Eat Stop Eat

An Effective Approach to Intermittent Fasting for a Rapid Weight Loss | the Secret to Burn Fat, Reset your Metabolism, and Heal your Body without Suffering Hunger

[Thomas Slow]

Legal & Disclaimer

The information contained in this book and its contents is not designed to replace or take the place of any form of medical or professional advice; and is not meant to replace the need for independent medical, financial, legal or other professional advice or services, as may be required. The content and information in this book has been provided for educational and entertainment purposes only.

The content and information contained in this book has been compiled from sources deemed reliable, and it is accurate to the best of the Author's knowledge, information and belief. However, the Author cannot guarantee its accuracy and validity and cannot be held liable for any errors and/or omissions. Further, changes are periodically made to this book as and when needed. Where appropriate and/or necessary, you must consult a professional (including but not limited to your doctor, attorney, financial advisor or such other professional advisor) before using any of the suggested remedies, techniques, or information in this book.

Upon using the contents and information contained in this book, you agree to hold harmless the Author from and

1

against any damages, costs, and expenses, including any legal fees potentially resulting from the application of any of the information provided by this book. This disclaimer applies to any loss, damages or injury caused by the use and application, whether directly or indirectly, of any advice or information presented, whether for breach of contract, tort, negligence, personal injury, criminal intent, or under any other cause of action.

You agree to accept all risks of using the information presented inside this book.

You agree that by continuing to read this book, where appropriate and/or necessary, you shall consult a professional (including but not limited to your doctor, attorney, or financial advisor or such other advisor as needed) before using any of the suggested remedies, techniques, or information in this book.

Table of Contents

INTRODUCTION

The Eat-Stop-Eat protocol is one of several intermittent fasting methods that have helped many people lose excess body weight and, in the process, improve their general health. It's also one of the most popular protocols because it's one of the simplest and most flexible of the current intermittent fasting protocols. And in this book, you will get the opportunity to learn what the protocol really is about, the science behind weight loss, and how to optimally implement this protocol.

The most important reason for intermittent fasting is weight loss. It aims to reduce energy intake by consuming less meals. However, weight loss is not possible if high-energy foods (processed foods, fatty / fried meats, fast food foods, various pastries, etc.) are involved during the eating period.

Chapter 1: Intermittent Fasting

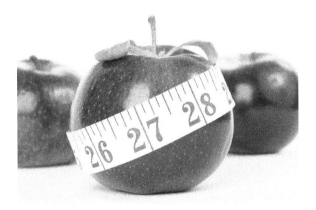

Definition

It is not the type or content of the food, but the diet in which the time zone of food is consumed. It is not a type of diet but a control of consumption time. Intermittent Fasting or Intermittent Fasting is the type of nutrition in which energy intake is restricted for a period of time and it is applied periodically.

During fasting, blood glucose decreases to very low levels 2-3 hours after the last eating. In this way, ketosis, the natural fat burning state, starts when the body lacks glucose. Ketosis; intermittent fasting is the cause of the body burning fat.

Studies have shown that intermittent fasting can support weight loss by helping to burn fat, help with metabolism, and the positive effects of this eating pattern on insulin resistance; It shows potential benefits like reducing inflammation, supporting a healthy digestive system. In this way, a nutritional model is associated with the level of ghrelin, which is known as the fasting hormone, and the level of saturation hormone leptin; it also changes insulin hormone levels. It decreases insulin, increases growth hormone levels and promotes norepinefrein secretion. Thanks to these changes, the metabolic rate can increase by 3.6-14%. The main reason for its success is that intermittent fasting generally helps to get fewer calories.

Scientific facts

How IF Affects the Body

When you're feeling hungry, your body is under the sway of two very important hormones: leptin and ghrelin, and Intermittent Fasting affects both of those hormones substantially. In a typical situation, leptin decreases sensations of being hungry, and ghrelin makes you feel hungry instead. While leptin is secreted from fat cells throughout the body, ghrelin is only secreted from the stomach's lining. Together, leptin and ghrelin communicate with the brain's hypothalamus, telling the body when to stop or start eating. During IF, these hormones are released less often, causing the body to have a whole different experience of hunger and fullness.

Another important hormone in the context of eating and hunger suppression is insulin itself. The pancreas produces insulin, and it regulates how much glucose exists in our blood. Ultimately, high or low amounts of insulin affect the individual's weight greatly. Too little insulin and one can't keep weight on. Too much insulin and one can't lose weight whatsoever. While it seems that lower insulin is desired, there has to be a healthy balance, for **too low** insulin is actually disastrous for the body since glucose (or blood sugar) is a large part of how the body gets energy.

One final influencer of the body's hunger and weight loss situation is the individual's thyroid. If the thyroid is overactive, metabolism will work quickly, and energy, health, and weight will be affected. Conversely, an underactive thyroid will slow metabolism, energy, and health, and it will contribute to increased weight.

In the end, Intermittent Fasting affects the individual's weight by varying the production of these three important hormones and by working with the thyroid's natural potential. Essentially, those practicing IF will trigger these hormones to be released less often (or more consistently if the person is obese or diabetic to start with) due to the less-frequent eating schedule. Eventually, even the thyroid's effects should become balanced out through this altered eating schedule.

IF and Diabetes

For people with diabetes, Intermittent Fasting poses certain risks as well as incredible benefits. People with diabetes have altered insulin levels compared to the non-diabetic person, due to insulin resistance in their bodies. People with Type 1 diabetes cannot make insulin. They need to take insulin daily to have the energy and vigor to live. People with Type 2 diabetes have bodies that don't produce much insulin or don't use that insulin well at all.

With these altered productions of insulin, the blood sugar levels of the body have no way to be regulated, meaning that there's more standing glucose in the blood at all times with no way for it to get into the cells to be used for natural and physical energy. This higher blood sugar level can cause additional problems for the individual over time, but there is no legitimate cure other than taking insulin daily.

Intermittent Fasting, however, can provide a temporary cure when applied correctly in the lives of diabetic individuals (whose diabetic conditions are not severe). When IF is done on a daily basis with just a few fasting hours a day, people with diabetes show improved weight, blood sugar levels, and standing glucose levels. These individuals are not recommended to skip entire meals or fast for days at a time. Also, is not recommended for these people to strictly diet while they're applying IF. Instead, it works better to make food portions smaller and to eat fewer snacks in between.

IF and Heart Health

Heart health is a complicated issue in today's world. We all want to be healthy and thrive, but the foods we eat and the activities we engage in often don't align with those goals, and those more immediate actions win out. In effect, many of our hearts aren't as healthy as they could be. Heart disease is still the biggest killer in the world to this day. However, the introduction of Intermittent Fasting into someone's lifestyle can greatly alter this potential, for it can reduce many risks associated with heart disease.

For example, recent studies done on animals have proved that the practice of Intermittent Fasting improves numerous risk factors for heart disease. Some of these improvements include lowered cholesterol, reduced inflammation in the body, balanced blood sugar levels, and lower blood pressure. Essentially, IF won't cure heart disease, but it will reduce several risk factors that may exist in one's body (with or without him or her knowing).

When it comes down to it, as long as one's Intermittent Fasting experience involves the reintroduction of electrolytes into the body, there's no potential harm posed to the heart whatsoever. There's only potential for growth, bolstering, and strengthening. However, without the right reintroduction of electrolytes, there **is** still the possibility of heart palpitations in individuals attempting IF. The heart needs electrolytes for its stability and efficacy, so as long as you drink a bit of salt with your water, your heart will only thank you!

IF and Aging

People love to talk about how Intermittent Fasting can reverse the effects of aging, and they're not wrong! The tricky part is elucidating the science behind the process they're referencing. The anti-aging potential tied up with Intermittent Fasting applies mostly to two things: 1) your brain and 2) your whole body, through what's called "autophagy."

Overall, Intermittent Fasting heals the body through its ability to rejuvenate the cells. With this restricted caloric intake due to eating schedule or timing, the body's cells can function with less limitation and confusion while producing more energy for the body to use. In effect, the cells function more efficiently while the body can burn more fat and take in more oxygen for the organs and blood, encouraging the individual to live longer with increased sensations of "youth."

About those two original examples, Intermittent Fasting has been proven 1) to keep the brain fit and agile. It improves overall cognitive function and memory capacity as well as cleverness, wit, and quick, clear thinking in the moment. Furthermore, Intermittent Fasting 2) keeps the cells fit and agile through autophagy (which is kickstarted by IF), where the cells are encouraged to clean themselves up and get rid of any "trash" that might be clogging up the works. By just restricting your eating schedule a little bit each day (or each week), you can find your brain power boosted and your body ready for anything.

IF and the Female Body

Intermittent Fasting requires a different technique than most diets do, which is why it's more often referred to as a lifestyle. Additionally, this variance means that the effects of IF on the female body are a little different than the effects of the standard diet. For instance, dieting will easily cause weight loss in most people, but IF is a little trickier and much less consistent for women especially.

The female body, being created with birthing potential, has specific needs that are altered through an Intermittent Fasting eating schedule. With less hormones being released (which tell women when they are hungry and full) there is less fat being stored in their bodies and less fertility when it comes to their later aims of reproducing. In combination with a strict diet that counts calories or restricts fats, Intermittent Fasting can be dangerous for women of all ages.

For women who still want to work with Intermittent Fasting, there's a lot of hope left for you! Just make sure to follow these four steps to ensure that you're doing it in the most healthy way for your body and your future children. First, make sure you're very connected to your body. You'll want to be very aware if something on the inside seems "off" or "wrong" (bodily, emotionally, and mentally), especially considering all that's at stake, hormonally and reproductively.

Second, make serious effort to be aware of your body's cycles and note when things go askew. Without the right awareness of your menstruation, you risk going a long time with an altered cycle. This alteration might not sound like a lot, but it can affect many different aspects of your body and your childrearing potential.

Third, please don't try to combine strict dieting and Intermittent Fasting. I know you want to be fit and strong and slim, but you still want to make sure you're getting enough fat and calories, considering what your body is able to do with these right amounts of fat and calories.

Fourth and finally, make sure you're also not exercising too ferociously while you first transition to Intermittent Fasting. If you've been trying IF as a lifestyle for a while, you're welcome to add fitness and exercise back into the mix, but it is really dangerous for the female body to combine two intense practices at once. I understand the urge to lose weight and be healthy, but you'll need to make sure you're not eliminating **too much** from your body at any given time.

Misconceptions of fasting

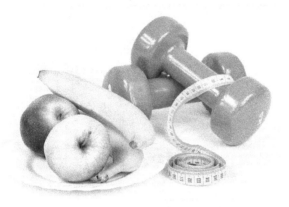

There's a lot of misinformation circulating about Intermittent Fasting, but the truth is out there, too! Here are 8 misconceptions about Intermittent Fasting and their respective **realities**.

It's not natural to fast like that.

BUSTED: It's more natural to practice Intermittent Fasting than it is to eat three full meals each day! It's more connected to our evolutionary drives and to our primitive selves to eat like this. And it's better for our brains, hearts, cells, and digestive systems to have a break from food once in a while to recalibrate. As you learned in the Introduction, people have been practicing Intermittent Fasting as long as humans have been in existence. It's only myths like this that circulate today that make it seem like IF is foreign, unhealthy, and dangerous. Animals of all types become healthier after periods of fasting, and humans are no different. Remember that we are animals and that IF is in our nature. Proceed with that confidence and knowledge!

There's only one way to do IF that's right and truly the best.

BUSTED: This myth is absolutely and utterly false. There is no one right way to practice Intermittent Fasting, and part of the beauty of IF is that there **are** so many different methods, meaning each approaching IF likely has a few different options to choose from. Similarly, different body and personality types will be drawn to different methods, based on individuals' abilities and goals. IF is about flexibility, adjustment, and self-correction. There's no one right method for everyone, and there's no "best" method to strive for. Do whatever method feels right and suits your life, and once you've found it, practice it as long as you can! That's far more realistic and accessible.

During fast periods, you literally can't eat anything.

BUSTED: This myth is partially true and partially false. It's true only for methods like 12:12, 14:10, 16:8, and 20:4 that require fasting and eating in alternation within each individual day. For 12:12 method, for example, you'd spend 12 hours fasting and 12 hours eating. In this case, you would definitely not eat anything or consume any calories during that 12-hour fasting window, but the same isn't true for methods that alternate between days "on" and days "off" between fasting and eating. For those types of methods, you absolutely can eat during fasting periods! It might feel counterintuitive as you read these words, but you don't explicitly have to eat **nothing** during fast periods. Most methods that have full days of fasting actually allow for caloric intake as long as it's restricted by 20-25% of one's normal intake. Therefore, for methods like 5:2, alternate-day, eat-stop-eat, and crescendo, on days when you're fasting, you can still consume around 500 calories, and that will help a lot!

You'll only gain weight if you try skipping meals.

BUSTED: This myth is based on the same logic that drives myth #3 about overeating. If you gorge yourself during your eating windows, you'll surely gain weight, but hardly anyone will continuously gorge with IF. Anyone who tries will realize how unsuccessful it is, so he or she will not **continuously** gorge in response. Anyone who doesn't realize his or her efforts with eating are unsuccessful will soon realize that something's wrong, as his or her weight shows no improvement. Skipping meals never **necessarily** means that someone will gain weight. It just means that people who skip meals **and gorge or overeat** when it **is** mealtime won't see the desired effects.

Your metabolism will slow down dangerously.

BUSTED: This myth is also addressed in chapter 12's Questions & Answers, but the point is that your metabolism won't slow down just because you're eating less often. People who think this myth is true, only assume that restricted caloric intake will make one's metabolism slow down over time, but these individuals forget that IF isn't **necessarily** about cutting down calories overall (although

19

methods like 20:4 don't leave much room for full caloric intake). It's actually about cutting down the **times** during which one consumes calories. There needn't be any caloric restriction whatsoever! It just depends on the practitioner and what he or she decides to do with dieting in addition to IF.

You'll almost assuredly overeat during eating windows, and that's not healthy at all.

BUSTED: While some people will have the **instinct** to overeat during eating windows, not everyone will overeat. Even those who do at the start will realize how to move forward without this overeating instinct in the future. Your body will urge you to overeat because, at the start, it won't realize what you're doing to it, but as long as you keep portion sizes largely the same and don't gorge on snacks, your body will adjust and so will your appetite.

You'll lose muscle in this endeavor.

BUSTED: This myth goes along the same lines as the first one, above. Just like your body won't enter the starvation mode (unless something goes very, very wrong or you're trying to do too much); your body won't lose muscle through IF. The only reason why IF **would** cause muscle loss would be if it was causing you to starve, but once again, the first myth addresses this falsity, making this myth false as well.

Your body will definitely enter in starvation mode.

BUSTED: Your body will **not** definitely enter in starvation mode through Intermittent Fasting. Skipping meals or adjusting to longer periods between meals where you don't eat is not going to make you starve. It's going to help your body remember how to absorb nutrients. It's going to help you thrive instead.

Is IF for you ?

As it turns out, Intermittent Fasting is simply not for everyone. Firstly, IF is not for a growing body, this is why children or teenagers should not participate in Intermittent Fasting on a daily basis; only up to 24 hours. You can imagine that a growing body needs all possible nutrients, and you can't achieve this with a decreased feeding window. If children or teenagers have to try Intermittent Fasting, they should only do it with the consent of a doctor.

Intermittent Fasting should be avoided by pregnant or breastfeeding women. Since these women need to feed for two persons, nutrient deprivation through Intermittent Fasting is really not indicated.

Starvation can also lead to reducing women's fertility, and since Intermittent Fasting may involve starvation, it should be avoided by women who are having difficulties to get pregnant. But this is just in the early phases of Intermittent Fasting, as training your mind and digestive system can help you not even feel hungry during a daily fasting program. IF done properly can rule out the hunger feeling, and can make women feel better about themselves and have increased energy levels. Bear in mind that women's hormones can be triggered by the following factors:

- not enough sleep, rest or recovery;

- too much stress;

- too much or too intense physical exercise;

- infections and inflammations, but also other diseases;

- poor food choices or less food.

Intermittent Fasting should not be tried by people suffering from diabetes who are using insulin. If you had a surgery or other medical intervention, you also need to forget about Intermittent Fasting during the recovery period. If you have a history of an eating disorder, then Intermittent Fasting is not for you. Anyone with a medical condition needs to get approval from their doctor before trying IF.

If you are wondering who can try Intermittent Fasting, then you only have to rule out children, teenagers, pregnant and breastfeeding women, or anyone suffering from a disease or medical condition that doesn't allow IF (according to a doctor).

Setting a Plan

It's nice to think of Intermittent Fasting as a way of life, so it's way beyond a diet. Why? Because it completely changes your life: the way you eat, when you eat, when it's the best time to exercise, plus, it has so many benefits (mentioned earlier in this book) that you can benefit from. It's quickly becoming one of the most interesting alternatives to the busy lifestyle of a modern human.

If you are struggling to do more tasks every working day (as it's all about better productivity nowadays), you probably don't have time for a proper lunch during your work, and perhaps everything is on the move. You might feel forced to try fast-food or to have unhealthy snacks at hand, but your schedule should not be an excuse for what you eat.

You need to be aware that fast-food has very low nutritional value and is definitely not healthy. But for some reason, it's consumed by most people nowadays because it's the cheapest food you can find out there and it's extremely fast to cook and serve. This is how the corporate lifestyle looks like, and it's very harmful to your body. On top of that, when you spend at least 12 hours at work and in traffic, getting a bit of free time of your own to cook your own meals sounds very complicated.

You need to take control of your life and to impose a schedule and diet that is healthier for you. This doesn't mean quitting your job (you still have bills to pay), but it means bringing some order into the chaos that is your lifestyle. How can you do that? Well, let's try to focus first on the food you eat. Eating nothing but burgers, pizzas, french fries, and chips will not do you any good for your general health. They have low nutritional value and too many calories. Plus having sodas or energy drinks is the poorest choice of drinks you can have with this food. So why not prepare your own food? Obviously, the fast-food chains don't care about your health, but you need to look after you. Head over to your local supermarket, look for fresh vegetables and fruits, dairy products and raw (but fresh) meat. Why not try some healthy oils into your diet? Forget about french fries, or other pre-cooked food, as you shouldn't use your microwave oven to cook your food.

Luckily for you, this book will also provide you some interesting recipes for you to try, so you don't have to panic as you don't know what to cook. You have a kitchen at home, use it! Perhaps doing your own shopping and cooking at home is more expensive than when you eat fast-food from different restaurants, but how much are you willing to pay extra when your health is at stake?

It's no shame to have your own lunch packed with you at work; this is food that you cooked for yourself, and you know exactly what it contains, and perhaps even how many calories it has. This might force you to radically change what you have in your refrigerator, so you need to get rid of any pre-cooked food, sodas or sweets that you might have in your refrigerator. Why not place in there vegetables, fruits, some dairy products and high quality proteins? If you normally buy chips, donuts, or other types of sweets or snacks, forget about them! It's time to eliminate them from your diet, as you should only try them on rare occasions. You need to replace them with fruits, as unlike the snacks mentioned previously, they can be a great source of minerals and vitamins.

Now that you've taken care of your nutrition, how about being less lazy and a lot more active? You may not have worked out during your lunch break, but you still need to start your day in an active way. Even if it's just a few ab crunches and push-ups, or something more complex like jogging, swimming, or working out at the gym - morning training is what you need to get your energy boost. However, I may be repeating myself, but I need to point this out: IT'S BETTER TO WORK OUT ON AN EMPTY STOMACH!

Different approaches

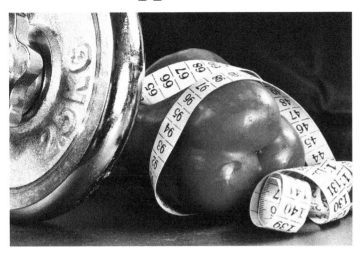

There are many approaches of intermittent fasting. In the end, the only one you should use is one that is going to work for you. Perhaps the hardest part about reaping the benefits of IF is that you are going to be hungrier than usual at the start. Stick with it! Sticking with IF may mean trying many different IF methods until you find one that you like. This doesn't mean finding an IF method that isn't any struggle at all, but rather finding an IF method that you know you can keep up with for whatever amount of time you've set as your goal. If your goal is to use IF to lose fat in 90 days, choose a plan that *you can stick with for 90 days*. It's as simple as that. With that in mind, let's discuss the main four IF methods: Leangains, Eat Stop Eat, The Warrior Diet, and Alternate Day Fasting. These methods are here because they're easy to understand, they have significant, proven benefits, and they're 100% free.

Alternate Day Fasting

Alternate Day Fasting is another simple yet demanding method that encourages more fat burning than easier methods. It may also be the hardest method to use. You just eat one day, and don't eat (or eat a small amount) the next.

How much you eat on your feeding days depends on your weight loss goals. In general women eat 2,000 calories on their feeding days and 400 calories on their fasting days. Men eat 2,500 calories on their feeding days and 500 on their fasting days. In general, if you can cut your calories by 20 to 35 percent of your regular intake on your feeding days, you can lose up to 2.5 pounds per week. I would highly recommend tailoring your calorie needs to your own lifestyle though. Remember, this can easily be done with a quick Google search where some 'calorie calculator' tools will appear on the first page. Lots of people, for whatever reason, are hesitant to count calories which is why I am constantly hounding you to do this.

Exercise is entirely up to you - this method focuses purely on eating. If you want an entirely neutral energy expenditure on your fasting day, it is possible to work out until you've lost the amount you plan to consume. For example, if you are somebody who wants to eat 500 calories on your fasting day, just jump on the treadmill for about an hour before you eat. This will balance out the low amount of calories consumed on a fasting day, and contribute towards weight loss.

The Warrior Diet

You could argue that The Warrior Diet is thousands of years old. Ori Hofmekler spent many years in the Israeli Defense Force and during this time he performed research on other soldiers' diets. This research extended to the dietary and training habits of ancient warriors, specifically Ancient Greeks and Romans. He published his first book on The Warrior Diet in 2002.

The entire diet bases itself around the sympathetic and parasympathetic nervous systems. By taking advantage of these systems, your body can utilize its nutrients to the fullest. During the day, your body spends energy using the sympathetic nervous system. During the night, your body replenishes that energy using the parasympathetic nervous system. For this reason, on The Warrior Diet, you have a non-feeding period of 18 hours during the day, and a 4 to 6 hour feeding period at night. During the feeding period at night, you consume only one large meal. The rule of thumb for this meal is that you stop eating once you want a drink (water) more than you want food.

While the 18 hours non-feeding period and 4 to 6 hour feeding period are the core concepts of this IF method, there are some added details about what you eat.

1. Do not eat processed foods, or foods that potentially contain added hormones

2. Do not drink alcohol

3. Eat carbohydrates last during your meal to maximize fat oxidation

Full body exercise is also a component of this IF method. It is encouraged that you work out during the 18-hour non-feeding period. This is supposed to simulate how prehistoric peoples (women included) had to hunt and fight while hungry.

IF should generally not be used if you are pregnant or under 18 years old and even more so here since this is a bit of a savage take on IF.

This diet is basically a step up from the 16:8 method. Once your body and mind become conditioned to that, this would be the logical next step. I do feel that the rule of thumb where you stop once you crave water more than food really is just a rule of thumb. If you're doing this for aesthetics, record your intake religiously.

Eat Stop Eat

Eat Stop Eat is an IF method developed by Brad Pilon. It's very simple; you have a non-feeding period of 24 hours once or twice a week. The rest of the week, you eat 'normally' ie. three square meals spread out over the day. Because of its simplicity, Eat Stop Eat is a great plan for people who don't like overthinking things or who have very hectic lifestyles. It is also a great plan for those coming off of an even more "powerful" IF method, such as Alternate Day Fasting. You also need to make sure that you do not have two 24 hour periods together in which you don't eat. For example, it would not be wise to eat only on the weekdays, and then eat nothing on the weekends. Instead, space the 24 hour periods out.

Leangains

Leangains aka "16:8" is an IF method created by Martin Berkhan. He is a nutritional consultant, writer, and personal trainer. He created the Leangains system specifically for his clients - but has shared it with the world as well. His system works best when you fine-tune it to your goals, but it can also be applied with just the basics. We will cover both.

There are two eating/non-eating periods. The non-feeding period lasts 16 hours. This closely follows 8 hours of eating time. Usually, during this 8-hour eating period you will consume your three daily meals. What you decide to eat for those meals depends entirely on your personal goals. Personally, I actually eat two very big meals as I find it extremely satisfying while still meeting my goal of either shedding some fat or maintaining a lean body.

If you are only interested in the broad picture, '16 hours fast, 8 hours eat' is all you need to know. We'll be going into some details now if you feel like you're up for a challenge. These can really maximise your results though more dedication is required.

Fasted Training

Fasted training works best for those who can work out on an empty stomach.

1. Begin workout, it lasts one hour

2. Immediately eat your largest meal of the day

3. Eat your second meal, fewer calories/carbs

4. Eat your third meal, even fewer calories/carbs

5. Begin your fast approximately 8 hours after you finished your workout

Early Morning Fasted Training

Early morning fasted training is for Berkhan's clients who prefer to work out as soon as they wake up, and then eat in the afternoon.

1. Work out for an hour as soon as you wake up (usually around 6 AM)

2. Take a zero calorie amino acid supplement (optional) 1 hour later

3. Take another zero calorie amino acid supplement 2 hours after that

4. Start the 8 hour feeding period (usually around noon)

5. Begin a 16 hour fasting period (usually at night before you sleep)

One Pre-Workout Meal

This is a protocol specifically for people with flexible working hours.

1. Eat the pre-workout meal (usually around noon) - this should be about 25% of your calorie goals

2. Work out sometime in the next few hours

3. Eat your largest meal of the day immediately afterward

4. Eat your smallest meal of the day a few hours later

5. Begin fasting approximately 8 hours after your first meal

Two Pre-Workout Meals

This is the best protocol to use if you have an average 9 to 5 job.

1. Eat the pre-workout meal (usually around noon) - this should be about 25% of your calorie goals

2. Eat your second meal before you go home, it should be the same size as the first

3. Work out for an hour once you get home

4. Eat the post workout meal, which should be your largest (about 60% of your calories)

5. Begin your 16 hours fast

As you can see, each of these protocols is just a different spin on the same idea: 16 hours non-feeding period, 8 hours feeding period. You can make your own so long as you stick to the key points. Some people even switch it to 14 hours fast, 10 hours eating if they find 16:8 too hard. I would say this is the most you can push it and realistically expect results though. It is important to note that your body should not ingest any calories while you are fasting. There are only a few things that are "ok" to swallow during the 16-hour non-feeding period. This includes water and black coffee. Zero calorie drinks should not be taken as they trigger your insulin response which tells your body 'let's hold onto this fat'. You are also allowed 1/2 to 1 teaspoon of milk per cup of coffee but use this sparingly. Up to 50 calories in the fasted period isn't too bad but ideally, you would only drink water during the 16-hour non-feeding period.

Fasting and Hormones

How Fasting Can Affect Your hormones and cells

As you fast, few things start to happen inside the body on the molecular and cellular levels. For instance, your body settles its hormone levels for making the stored fats easily accessible. Also, the cells begin the vital repair processes and alter the formation of genes.

Following are some changes which happen in the body during the fasting:

Insulin:

the sensitivity for insulin get enhanced, and the amount of insulin decreases dramatically. The low levels of insulin can make the stored fats of the body easily accessible for you.

Human growth hormone:

the level of the growth hormone increases drastically in your body, rising as high as 3-fold. It has advantages for muscular gain and fat loss, to mention a few. Cellular repair:

while fasting, the cells begin the cellular repair procedures. It includes autophagy, in which cells get digested and eliminate the dysfunctional and old protein, which made up inside the cells.

Gene expression:

there can be some changes within the functioning of genes about the protection from diseases and longevity. Such changes in the hormone level, gene expression, and cellular functioning are responsible for the benefits of health during intermittent fasting.

Chapter 2: Eat-Stop-Eat

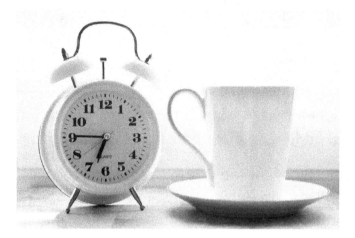

What is eat stop eat

The Eat Stop Eat is not a daily fasting program, in fact, it mostly encourages you to fast just once per week. The fasting period, in this case, would be just 24 hours, which might sound a bit scary for some of you out there, but hear me out! How about if you had just one whole day of fast per week, and the rest of the week you can regularly? Can you cope with this program? The 24 hour fast is one of the most popular programs practiced by different people worldwide. It was developed by Brad Pilon who had the bright idea to name this program very simple: Eat Stop Eat.

There are plenty of specialists and people who can agree that this program is the easiest one, and perhaps it should be the first Intermittent Fasting program to be tried by beginners. Some people might be thinking of trying more IF programs, but you need to ease into Intermittent Fasting; to take it slow because you will be able to deal a lot easier with possible symptoms like hunger, headaches, and dizziness. The Eat Stop Eat program is perhaps the most accessible and popular method for most Intermittent Fasting enthusiasts. Some people just like to fast completely for one day per week, every once in a while. Others are more ambitious and might want to try the 24 hours fast twice or three times a week. After all, it all depends on what you are looking to achieve. The beauty of this program is that it doesn't require any scheduling or special rules. You only have one rule: choose the day you want to fast! That's it!

Just like any other Intermittent Fasting program, this one doesn't mention anything about a special meal plan, you can eat whatever you want, as long as you respect the only rule that you have. Let's say that you like to hang out with your friends or family during weekends, have copious meals, and then you just want to fit in your favorite pair of jeans. In this case, I would strongly recommend having the fasting day on Tuesday or Wednesday, as you might not be able to have it on Monday (you are used to so much food during the weekend, so completely eliminating the food on Monday may be a bit too radical).

However, if you plan to try this program (or any Intermittent Fasting), you might need to take it easy with the calorie intake, as you probably want to lose some weight, or even to experience some other health benefits of Intermittent Fasting.

How to fast with eat-stop-eat style

Keep in mind that a significant portion of your daily liquid intake comes from the water in the food you eat, and since you're not eating when your fasting, it is advisable to drink a little more than you normally would.

Try your best to keep your calories as close to zero as possible. Once you start adding a "little bit" of cream and sugar to your coffee, or a "little sip" here or there you may find that your calorie intake slowly starts to creep up during your fast. Do your best to try and have a "zero tolerance approach" during your fast. When it comes to what else you can eat during your fasts, follow this guideline—guideline—the true benefit is learning to take breaks from eating, not to figure out how to "game the system."

I often get questions about consuming a "little bit" of beef broth, or coconut water, or xylitol, or other almost calorie-free foods during a fast. There is not enough research for me to answer questions on the metabolic effect of a small amount of calories from all the different food and ingredient sources. So, remember that calorie-free beverages are okay during your fasts, and calorie-free gum is all right in moderation, but try to avoid any other almost calorie-free foods. The key is to learn to take a break from eating, not to continue to reinforce the pattern of always eating and always being fed.

So, when it comes to what you can and cannot eat while fasting, follow this simple guideline: If you can go without then go without, but if you really can't go without then don't.

Avoid the mistakes of trying to fit as many fasts into a week as possible, or trying to extend your fasts far beyond 24 hours. As I mentioned earlier, I have found that 24-hours once or twice a week is the most flexible and convenient way to fast.

Extending beyond this greatly reduces the flexibility of Eat Stop Eat and may lead to a sort of "fasting burnout." Forcing yourself to fast too often or for too long to the point where you are dreading your next fast completely defeats the purpose of the Eat Stop Eat lifestyle.

The same goes for fasting more often, the benefits of fasting don't only come just from the time you are fasting, but also the time after the fast. Just like with exercise, there needs to be recovery time for you to get the full effects. That's why I recommend at least 48-hours of time in between each 24-hour fast.

After talking with literally hundreds of people who have been following Eat Stop Eat, I have noticed that the people who stay flexible and relaxed see the best weight loss results and are the most able to keep the weight off. On the other hand, the people who try to speed up the process by fasting multiple times per week or extending their fasts to 48 or even 72-hours do see quick results, but also "burn out" very quickly.

This is in agreement with the large volume of research on restrained eating, which eloquently shows that the more restrained a person is with their eating, meaning the more rules they try and follow (good food/ bad food lists, food combining, etc.) the more likely they will see quick weight loss, but also the more likely they will experience extreme weight rebounds after they have broken some of their rules and restraints.

Under similar conditions, the more restrained you are with your fasts, the more likely you will feel guilty if you break your rules and end up overeating. The bottom line is that the Eat Stop Eat lifestyle should free you from obsessive-compulsive eating, but this should not be at the expense of simply learning to obsess about your fasting.

The same "fasting burnout" happens to people who combine fasting with strict dieting, or excessive amount of exercise. As a general rule of thumb, if you are having difficulties organizing fasting, exercising, and dieting into your schedule you are most likely doing too much of at least one of these activities.

Consider fasting the easiest way possible to get results. Essentially you are getting results from doing nothing, so you do not need to make it any more complicated than an occasional break from eating, but you should go out of your way to view every single complete fast as a "mini-victory"— positive reinforcement at its finest.

You can say goodbye to obsessing over your daily calorie intake, over obsessing over how many carbs you ingested today.

You can say goodbye to extremely restrictive bans on foods as well as on other forced behaviors in pursuance of focusing on getting back into shape in a healthy, natural way by following your body's biology.

You have probably blamed yourself, or your lack of self-discipline in the past. You probably have blamed calories and your dieting formulas which most certainly did not bring anything good your way.

The truth is that there is no one and nothing to blame here. Every step you have taken in the past can teach you something which will help you to succeed in the future.

Another truth is that losing weight can be an extremely difficult thing to do and there are several different reasons behind this.

If you are focused on the weight loss industry, you have probably been told many times before how easy it is to shed those additional pounds.

The industry generally suggests you take this pill, drink that beverage or buy this equipment and simply enjoy your additional pounds melting on their own.

The truth is that the industry generates billions of dollars every year thanks to individuals who spend their money on different weight loss tools and products which can only be effective in the short-run.

Accordingly, many people struggling with weight are still overweight despite hundreds of dollars spent in the industry.

Now, you probably wonder why it is so hard and challenging to lose those additional pounds. It should be noted that there is no magical pill, magical tool or magical equipment that can make the process runs smoothly.

Dieting plans which suggest you completely change your dieting pattern, quit eating your favorite foods and similar restrictions do not work.

There is also scientific evidence as clear as it can get that suggests that cutting your daily calorie intake will not by any means lead to health gains or long-term weight loss.

It would be logical that most dieters have realized they have wrong dieting patterns, but still, individuals set those same weight goals every year.

The truth is that dieting failures are the norm. There is also a massive stigma surrounding heavier people and on many occasions, we can witness the massive blame game which is directed towards dieters who are not able to shed those additional pounds.

On the other hand, looking from a scientific point of view, it is clear that dieting most certainly sets up a truly unfair fight.

Many people are confused to learn that dieting plans suggesting extreme dieting changes, but that this only comes as a result of the statements does not square with their previous observations.

There are some thin people who consume junk food and still stay thin without their food choices affecting their weight.

These people most usually think that they stay in shape due to their dieting habits, but the truth is that genetics plays a massive role in helping them stay fit.

These people are praised over their dieting choices as others can only see what they consume, but they cannot examine what is inside their genes.

Why no longer fast?

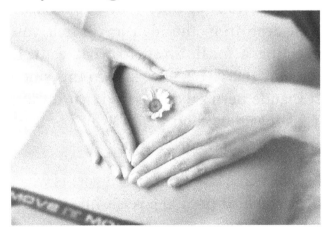

There are reasons that I prefer 24-hour fasts over longer fasts. One is the ease and simplicity of 24-hour fasts; another is that they allow people to still eat every day. I also believe the goal should be to balance the times spent fed and fasted, rather than to completely remove eating for days on end.

To understand the main reason why I do not promote the idea of longer fasts I'm going to need to introduce you to the reciprocal relationship that exists in your body between your fat burning metabolism and your carbohydrate burning metabolism. In order to meet the energy requirements of an average day, your body will burn a blend of carbohydrates and fats. In the resting state (not exercising), this blend will largely be determined by the blend of carbohydrates and fats in your diet. As you gradually start to enter the fasted state, this blend will slowly favor fat over carbohydrates, and this is for good reason.

When you fast for short periods of time your blood sugar remains stable. It will drop from the high levels that you typically have after eating a meal, down to what we call fasted levels and then stay there. We have known this since 1855, when scientist Claude Bernard discovered that during the initial stages of fasting, the blood sugar level was kept normal due to the breakdown of the liver glycogen.

Liver glycogen (the sugar being stored in your liver) is what keeps your blood sugar stable at normal levels while you are fasting for short periods of time.

However, if you keep fasting eventually you liver glycogen will begin to run out, and other compensatory mechanisms must come in to play to maintain your blood sugar levels.

As you fast, you slowly enter fasted state metabolism— a metabolism based around mobilizing and using your body fat as a fuel. Fasted state metabolism is a fat-burning metabolism— using fat (and later ketones) as a fuel in order to preserve your blood sugar levels and your body protein stores. This is true during short 12 to 24-hour fasts and much longer fasts.

The longer you fast, the greater the alterations that must be made to ensure that you are able to burn as much fat as possible. In short, the longer your fast, the more fat burning dominates carbohydrate burning. Once you are this far into fat burning, you simply cannot turn it off like a switch when you start eating again. And this is where some of the scare about longer term fasting comes from. Specifically, an increase in blood free fatty acid levels is well known to push your muscles towards oxidizing a high amount of fat as a fuel, but in doing so it must also inhibit glucose oxidation. This change begins very early during a fast, as early as the 8 to 10-hour mark, and then gradually progresses as the level of free fatty acids build up in your blood and the level of glycogen decreases in your liver.

There is no real way around this. If you want your muscles to burn your body fat as a fuel, then you can't have your muscles also burn high amounts of carbohydrates. And since your muscles are not oxidizing carbohydrates, less glucose is actually entering your muscles. It's still in your blood, but your muscles don't want any. They are "full" from a carbohydrate point of view— there would be no place to put the glucose if it entered your muscles.

As a result, it is a well-established fact that longer periods of fasting (48 to 72-hours and beyond) not only induce a high level of fat oxidation, but also create a short period of insulin resistance at the muscular level in the immediate hours after the fast is finished.

Now, this doesn't happen during a 24-hour fast as it takes around 24-hours just to deplete liver glycogen levels, but once glycogen has been depleted and the levels of fat in your blood are increased, changes start to occur to ensure that your blood sugar levels still remain stable, even in the face of diminished glycogen stores. This seems to happen earlier in women than in men, possibly due to the fact that women have higher levels of fat in their blood and a better ability to burn fat while in the fasted state. Basically, women enter fasted state metabolism quicker than men.

So, when you fast for extended periods (two to three days and beyond) your body goes into a kind of permanent fat burning physiology which involves a down regulation of the hormones and enzymes responsible for carbohydrate burning.

Normally, this isn't an issue since during short fasts we start to enter the fasted state and increase the amount of fat we burn, but we begin eating again before the body can compensate for these maintained elevations in fat burning by decreasing insulin sensitivity.

However, when you greatly pass 24-hours of fasting by 2 to 3-fold, this decreased sensitivity to insulin can build up and carry over to when you are eating. Towards the end of longer-term fasts your body will release far more fat into your bloodstream than you can actually use without adding in some form of exercise. So, even though you've ended your fast and had a meal, it's not as if all of those FFA that were released from your body fat stores suddenly vanish— they need some time to either be burned as a fuel, or restored as body fat.

Now, if for some reason all of these changes were to immediately reverse after your first bite of a meal after your fast, you would experience some very nasty consequences. Firstly, you'd risk becoming hypoglycemic; you'd also have an extremely high fat level in your blood with no way to get rid of that fat, except to re- store it all immediately as body fat. Neither one of these are ideal situations and for these reasons it takes your body a period of time (several hours) to come back into a normal state with normal levels of insulin sensitivity after longer fasts.

In fact, fasting for 72-hours can temporarily blunt insulin's ability to prevent lipolysis even in the fed state. This illustrates the transition state that occurs after a longer fast. The elevated levels of growth hormone that are released into your blood following a longer-term fast does not vanish the minute you take a bite of your first meal, and can actually take several hours to come back down to non-fasting levels.

So just as you "ramp up" into fat burning mode in a fast, you also have to "ramp down" at the end of a fast. However, it's also been found that after this acute period of insulin resistance your body may actually return to a level of improved insulin sensitivity— as periods of longer fasting are associated with improvements in insulin sensitivity when measured several days later.

The bottom line is that there is a major switch from glucose oxidation to fatty acid oxidation that occurs during fasting, and this switch needs some time to become apparent. What may be less obvious is that this switch requires a similar duration of time to be undone when refeeding commences. In other words, there is a gradual transition into fasted state metabolism and there is a gradual transition back into fed state metabolism. Finally, the longer the time spent in the fasted state, the longer it takes to return to the fed state.

In the end, I'm not sure how short periods of acute insulin resistance affect human health, some people have even argued that they are good for long-term health and anti-aging.

These are just some of the reasons why Eat Stop Eat is based around brief 24-hour periods of fasting. There is ease and flexibility associated with 24-hours of fasting divided between two days, but this ease and flexibility is erased when you begin to fast for longer periods of time.

What to do while fasting

Since I do not consider the Eat Stop Eat lifestyle to be a diet, it would be a waste for me to fill two hundred pages of this book with recipes, food combining instructions or calorie and protein charts (go browse through any other diet book and you'll quickly discover that most of the pages are just that).

Doing so would not help you in any extra capacity. In fact, it would do quite the opposite. It would clutter your mind with needless rules to obsess and stress over, and possibly set you up for disinhibition effect while not moving you any closer to your weight loss goals. Instead, the best thing I can do is provide you some tips to help make your fasts a little easier.

In the morning start your day with a large glass of water. Black coffee and tea are also allowed during a fast. You may also find diet colas useful, and don't worry about having a small amount of artificial sweeteners during your fast, in my opinion the health benefits of fasting far outweigh any worry about the small and infrequent intake of artificial sweeteners.

Also, the current buzz about aspartame causing giant insulin spikes is not founded in science. There have been multiple studies on aspartame and its effect on insulin and growth hormone and they have all found no negative effects on either hormone.[

The other common misconception about coffee, teas, and colas is that caffeine causes giant increases in insulin. While it is true that caffeine can cause an increased insulin response to large doses of carbohydrates (caffeine + carbs = more insulin release than carbs alone),[245],[246] I have never seen any research suggesting that caffeine alone, without any carbs, causes insulin release. From a metabolic point of view, these drinks should not interfere with your fasts. This being said, try to keep your coffee and tea consumption to roughly what it would be on the days you are not fasting. Remember fasting should not be an excuse to drastically alter how you eat or drink.

Food is a form of bio-feedback. It is a form of stimulus in our everyday lives. So, when parts of our days are lacking excitement or stimulation (like when we are sitting in a car stuck in rush hour traffic), we seek stimulation in the form of foods and snacks.

Have you ever had a really boring day at work? Did you ever notice how often you snacked, or made coffee? This is because you are replacing mental stimulation with food stimulation.

A little complex, but it is the short answer to why we should stay busy while fasting. Other than staying busy, you can go about your day as if it were any other day. You can go to work, go shopping, go work out. Whatever it is you normally do during your day.

In fact, you will probably find that you have a lot of spare time on your fasting day. Almost everyone who lives the Eat Stop Eat lifestyle experiences this new freedom and extra

49

time. At this moment, you will also realize how much of your daily routine is spent planning, preparing, going out for, and eating food.

Taking a break from eating might just be the only way to actually free up useful time in your week.

Lastly, view every single fast you complete as a small win towards your weight loss goals. This is a unique feature that sets fasting apart from traditional dieting. By viewing each fast as a small win, you create a positive reinforcement as you move towards your weight loss goals. By conquering a fast you teach yourself that weight loss is possible, and that YOU are in control.

The main problem with traditional diets is that they seem like a long, slow march towards an inevitable failure. For example, going weeks and weeks without messing up or cheating only to hit that one day where you break and eat a donut. This only teaches you that you will inevitably fail at dieting; this negative reinforcement can destroy your future weight loss goals.

Stay positive and flexible with fasting. Every single 24-hour fast you complete is small win towards hitting your weight loss goals.

Tips to succeed

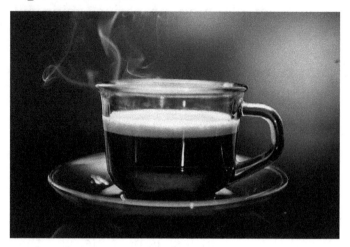

A Clear and Compelling Reason

Why do you want to fast intermittently using the Eat-Stop-Eat diet? Unless you're clear about it and unless it's compelling, I'm afraid your chances of succeeding are low. Why?

With a clear and compelling reason, you'll have enough motivation to stay the course even when the going gets really tough. If your reason for doing the Eat-Stop-Eat is shallow or flimsy, your chances of quitting after your 1st or 2nd 24-hour fasting day will be very, very high.

While losing weight and looking/ feeling great are valid reasons for doing the Eat-Stop-Eat protocol, those aren't very compelling reasons. To clarify your compelling reason for doing the protocol, ask "Why" until it's no longer possible to ask the question.

For example, you want to lose weight, so you decide to get into the Eat-Stop-Eat protocol. Why do you want to lose weight? If that's your end goal, I'm sorry, but it will not get you through when things get tough in the Eat-Stop-Eat diet. But if the reason you want to lose weight is to bring your health risks down and be as healthy as you can be, ask yourself why health is that important to you? Some sensible answers include:

– Because you want to see your children grow up to be adults and have their own children too;

– Because you don't want your wife to get widowed early and be lonely for the rest of her life; and

– Because you don't want to die a slow and painful death due to debilitating diseases like cancer, diabetes, or heart problems.

Having clear and compelling reasons like these will make you feel that the challenges and sacrifices you'll need to make on the Eat-Stop-Eat protocol will be worth it. And when you feel that way, you can power through the difficult stages of the protocol.

Feed Before the Fast

I'm not talking about eating food but feeding your mind prior to fasting so you can be in the right mindset and be optimally prepared when you finally take action. What does feeding the mind prior to the actual implementation of the Eat-Stop-Eat protocol look like? Here are some ideas:

– Read books, blogs, or articles and watch vlogs about the Eat-Stop-Eat method; and – If you know people who have successfully accomplished their weight and health goals via the protocol or intermittent fasting in general, reach out to them so you can have reasonable expectations about your up-and-coming Eat-Stop-Eat journey.

By getting enough experiential information about Eat-Stop-Eat, you can prepare yourself well.

Build Up Your Fasting Endurance

One of the reasons why many people drop out of the intermittent fasting game, in general, is hitting the ground running at full throttle. By this, I mean they try to fast for 20 to 24 hours immediately without giving their bodies and minds the chance to adjust to such a rigorous practice. Going without food for 20 to 24 hours straight isn't something to be taken lightly.

Can you imagine Usain Bolt, the fastest man in sprinting history, sprinting at maximum speed directly after getting up from bed in the morning? Stupid, right? He won't be able to run at top speed straight from waking up and worse, he can tear a muscle or ligament by going all out without the benefit of warming up and limbering his leg muscles.

It's the same with intermittent fasting, particularly for protocols like the Eat-Stop-Eat, which require 24-hour fasts. It's not something ordinary humans can do.

Hence, it can be very, very hard or even impossible for a beginner to successfully complete a 24-hour fast straight out of the gate.

A very good starting point is your average nightly sleeping hours. Let's say you sleep an average of 8 hours nightly. That's already 8 hours of fasting. If you take breakfast within 30 minutes upon waking up and if you eat your last meal of the day 1 hour before bed, it means you're already fasting for 9 ½ hours nightly on average. Let that be your baseline.

Start by adding an hour or two to your baseline by delaying your breakfast. If you delay your breakfast by an hour, or 1 ½ hours after waking up, you extend your fasting endurance to 10 ½ hours already. If you normally skip breakfast and go straight to lunch, then you're already fasting for over 12 hours every day. Gradually delay your first meal of the day by 1 hour every week or two or eat your last meal 1 hour earlier than you normally would every week or two. By doing that, you can gradually build up your fasting endurance.

Plan Your Fasting Days

Because you'll have no access to calories on your fasting days, it's best to schedule them on your least physically but non-consecutive busy days, especially if you'll schedule your steady state cardio exercises on those days. But if you're the type of person who finds it easier to diet during your busiest days of the week because your mind's preoccupied with a lot of things, you can schedule it on 2 of your busiest days of the week.

Work on Your Mental Barriers

Most of the concerns about fasting are mental, except in situations when a person is experiencing real physiological and physical danger during a very severe fast. Many people have already disqualified themselves from fasting even before giving it a shot by thinking, "I'm not built for it" or "I can't control my appetite." In other words, many people aren't able to fast intermittently simply because they've already decided in their minds that they can't do it.

Here's something to – pardon the pun – chew on as you contemplate on the Eat-Stop-Eat protocol: People of average weight can live without food for up to 40 days. That's 40 frickin' days! With the Eat-Stop-Eat, you'll only need to fast 2 days a week. And it's not even 2 straight days because you should fast on 2 non-consecutive days.

Many times, the hunger that we feel are either mental or a simple case of dehydration, in which case drinking a glass or two of water is enough to quell hunger pangs. Unless you have a pre-existing medical condition that can be aggravated by fasting regularly, there's very little reason to believe that you can't succeed at intermittent fasting.

When you think about it, physical barriers are easier to dismantle or breakthrough than mental ones. And one of the best ways to gradually break down mental barriers to intermittent fasting is by increasing one's knowledge about it. In particular, a highly recommended resource is the book Eat-Stop-Eat by no less than the man himself, Brad Pilon.

Don't Broadcast It

Next, to your mental barriers, the next biggest obstacles are the people around you, particularly their negative reactions and potentially discouraging words. This shouldn't be a surprise, especially from your family members. They will probably be critical of your Eat-Stop-Eating plans because of 2 things: genuine concern for you and ignorance of intermittent fasting. Hence, you must do your best to not let other people know what you're doing unless they've already done intermittent fasting or are knowledgeable about its health-related benefits.

Keep Hunger at Bay

If you are following the 5: 2 diet, then you will be restricting your calorie intake on the fast days. One of the major reasons why a lot of dieters give up on their diets is because of hunger. If you learn to keep your hunger pangs at bay, it will become easier to stick to the diet. Also, by understanding your hunger cues, you can differentiate between real and psychological hunger. Instead of eating whenever you think you are hungry, you will learn to eat only when your body needs to eat. Hunger pangs are quite common during the first couple of weeks of fasting when your body is getting used to the calorie restriction. In this section, you will learn about the different tips you can follow to keep hunger pangs at bay.

You must ensure that you are keeping your body hydrated always. Dehydration can make you feel quite tired and even cause a headache. Also, the best way to curb hunger is by drinking water.

Whenever you experience a hunger pang, drink a glass of water, give yourself twenty minutes, and the hunger pang will pass. At times, you might think you are hungry, but it might just be thirst. So, staying hydrated while fasting will improve your overall health and help you control your hunger too. Whenever a hunger pang strikes you, it can be difficult to focus on anything other than the hunger pangs. The best thing to do at such times is to remind yourself of the reasons why you started the diet. You might want to improve your overall health or might want to lose weight. Regardless of your reasons for dieting, it is a good idea to remind yourself of the same. You can make a list of all the reasons why you want to diet and glance at the list whenever you feel like giving in to any unhealthy cravings.

Coffee is one of the best ways to curb hunger pangs. If you are used to drinking coffee as soon as you wake up in the morning, then it will give you the necessary energy to keep going until lunchtime. You can substitute coffee with tea too. However, you cannot add any milk or sugar to these beverages since it will only increase your calorie intake. Try to stick to herbal teas and black coffee.

You can distract yourself from thinking about food by focusing on activities you like or even your work. When you occupy yourself with work, you will not have the time to think about food or hunger. Have there been times when you were so engrossed with the work that you forgot to eat? Well, you will essentially be trying to recreate this scenario. All protocols of intermittent fasting tend to free up a lot of your time, and you can use this time to work on things you love. If you have a hobby you enjoy, then go ahead and spend some time on it. By staying productive, you can prevent your mind from thinking about food.

Focusing on your dental hygiene is another way to ensure that you complete your fast. Having fresh and minty breath tends to reduce your desire to eat. On the fast days, after you eat a meal or a snack, don't forget to brush your teeth quickly. It is a way to signal your mind that you are done eating. It will not only improve your oral health but will help keep those cravings in check.

Don't take a lot of stress and learn to keep calm. When you are under stress, your body releases cortisol, a stress-inducing hormone that increases your desire to eat. The more stressed you are, the greater will be your desire to eat. Learning to control your stress has other health benefits like stabilizing your blood pressure and improving your ability to sleep. Apart from this, it also helps with better decision making and gives you mental clarity. So, by learning to control stress, it will not only help curb hunger pangs but will improve your overall health too. Try to spend some time outdoors, talk to a friend, spend time with your loved ones, or do anything else that will make you feel calm and relaxed.

Whenever you eat, you must ensure that your meals are rich in protein, fiber, and naturally fatty food. When you consume nutrient-dense foods, it helps you feel fuller for longer. Not just that, but it also provides your body with all the nutrients it needs.

On the days of the fast, make sure that you don't just slouch on your couch all day long. When your mind is idle, it tends to start thinking. So, get on with your day and move around a little. Don't opt for a sedentary lifestyle if you want to be able to stick to this diet.

There is another simple way to curb hunger, and that's by chewing gum. The chewing motion helps trick your mind into thinking you are full and helps keep hunger at bay.

Stay Motivated

At times, it can become rather difficult to stick to the diet. You might be surrounded by plenty of temptations, or you might even feel disheartened.

Regardless of the reason, here are three simple tips you can use to ensure that your motivation levels don't falter while dieting.

The first thing you must do is start using the mirror instead of a weighing scale to gauge your progress. When you get started with the diet, stand in front of a full-length mirror and look at all the areas in your body you want to lose weight from. If you want, you can take a picture of yourself. As you continue to follow the diet, there might be times when the diet works, but you cannot see a change in the weighing scales. If that's the case, then use the picture to see the improvement. You might not notice a sudden dip in the scales, but after a couple of weeks, you can see a positive change in your body measurements.

It is also a good idea to start a diet with a partner. You can team up with a friend, family member, colleague, or even your spouse. Going through a diet when you have someone to keep you company makes things easier. Not just that, you will also have a support system in place. You can fast, exercise, shop for groceries, and plan the meals together. Whenever you feel like giving up, you will have someone to help you stay on track and keep going.

You must make it a point to include different foods to your diet. If you keep eating the same items daily, you will certainly get bored. It is quintessential to ensure that your diet doesn't get repetitive or boring. Make a meal plan for all the fasting and non-fasting days, look for healthy recipes online, and stock up your pantry with the necessary ingredients.

Combining keto

Without a doubt, the Ketogenic Diet (popularly known as the Keto Diet) has gained a lot of popularity over the past years. You have probably heard of it already, as everybody is talking about it, since the Keto Diet proved to be one of the most effective programs for health management and weight loss.

This diet is a method to reprogram your body to burn fat for energy, instead of using the glucose from carbs or other sources. If Intermittent Fasting has the approach of restraining yourself from eating for a while, the Keto Diet suggests something different to have this outcome (the fat burning process). It suggests to revolutionize your meal plan, change it radically, to literally eat more fats and only a few carbs (and if possible, to avoid them at all).

When we stuff our faces with processed food (the main source of carbs), it's no wonder that our bodies have a "default fuel type" (glucose). The energy resulted from glucose is used by the whole body (including the brain), and it's vital for the body to function properly. The big problem with glucose is that this energy source is not quite "green," so it's harmful to the environment (your body). Why? Because it gets stored (if not burnt) in your blood, and this can be the beginning of your health problems.

Therefore, we do know what's causing our health issues (a very high volume of carbs). Now, the real question is what to do about it? How can we reverse this process (the increase of blood sugar level)? If we are more active, we will probably burn a lot more glucose than we normally do, so there will not be too much glucose going for your blood. However, why do we have to be so addicted to carbs? Can't we replace them with some other macronutrients?

Well, this is what the Keto Diet is designed to do. To change the way you eat, and completely replace the glucose (as your default energy source), with fats.

You will be amazed at how quickly your body can adapt to the latest changes. Imagine this scenario: your body can't find any more glucose to burn, so it has to look for alternative energy sources. If you are so used to eating plenty of carbs, this is the moment when your body is craving for more carbs. However, you must take control of the situation, and instead of feeding your body carbs, you must feed it something else a lot less harmful, in order to have a different fuel type, something more "eco-friendly."

As it turns out, fats can easily replace carbs in your diet, but your body needs to adapt and to find a way to get energy from fats. This is when the metabolic state of ketosis kicks in, as your blood sugar and insulin levels are decreasing, the ketone level is increasing. Your body will use ketones to break through the fat tissue, and fatty acids, to release the energy stored in there. Released by the liver, ketones are essential for the metabolic state of ketosis.

You probably have figured it out for yourself, the Keto Diet is yet another LCHF example; perhaps the most popular one. The regular western diet, full of fast-food and other examples of processed food, is simply packed with carbs. It's really pointless to find out the exact ratio for such meals, but in some cases, the carbs intake can represent around 70%, which is way too much for your body to process. The Keto Diet comes with a different approach, though. It suggests a ratio of 65% - 75% fats, and only 5% - 15% carbs (or none at all), while the rest is supposed to be proteins.

The biggest controversy here is how can you possibly eat so much fat and get slimmer? Well, as you know, calories are burned through physical exercise, and burning calories will get you energized. Fatty food doesn't have to be a calorie bomb; you can still eat this type of food and seriously decrease the number of calories you consume. So yes, the Keto Diet involves eating less food as well, but a lot healthier. As your body literally now runs on fats, it will have no difficulties in burning fats, whether it's the fat you eat or what is stored in your fat tissue. You can't wish for a better combination than to have Intermittent Fasting and the Keto Diet together in order to lose weight and to improve your overall health.

These two are so compatible together, you can experience the full benefits of them. Speaking of benefits, you are probably wondering what are the benefits of the keto diet. Obviously, this diet has a positive impact on people with pre-diabetes or diabetes. When you almost completely eliminate the glucose from your diet, your blood sugar and insulin levels will decrease. This can only prevent or reverse pre-diabetes of diabetes. When people need insulin to treat their diabetes, the keto diet can't make too much of a difference, but there are people suffering from diabetes, who were able to quit their treatment after trying the keto diet for a while. Again, make sure that you work with a physician, if you are diabetic and using insulin to help regulate your blood sugar levels.

When it comes to diseases or other medical conditions, the ketogenic diet has plenty of other benefits, as you can see below:

- heart disease. Since the keto diet seriously impacts your blood sugar, blood pressure and cholesterol levels, so indirectly, the keto diet can prevent any risks of heart disease;

- cancer. You are probably aware that cancer can be caused by the food we eat. Well, the keto diet is here to help, as all of its ingredients are extremely healthy. Plus, the keto diet (and Intermittent Fasting also) can trigger Autophagy, a process that can track down, repair or replace any damaged intracellular components, including the ones from cancer cells. Therefore, the keto diet has a role to play in preventing cancer or even reversing cancer in an incipient phase.

 - Parkinson's and Alzheimer's disease. Not surprisingly, this diet can improve cognitive and mental function, so it can prevent or slow down the progression of neurodegenerative diseases, such as Alzheimer's or Parkinson's disease;

- epilepsy. There are some studies proving that the Keto Diet can reduce seizures in epileptic children and adults;

- brain injuries. It looks like this diet can have a positive impact on reducing the effects of concussions, and the recovery time after a brain injury;

- polycystic ovarian syndrome. Studies have shown that polycystic ovarian syndrome can be caused by high insulin levels. As you already know, this meal plan significantly reduces those insulin levels;

- acne can be caused by too much glucose. Well, since this diet lowers the glucose level from your body, it also has a major impact on acne, but also on other skin conditions.

Unlike many other harsh diets, the ketogenic diet can be easily practiced by most people; it doesn't involve too many restrictions, but it requires you to radically change what you eat. The keto grocery list would include: broccoli, cauliflower, mushrooms, eggs, avocado, sardines, pickles, different types of seeds (sunflower, pumpkin), pecans, olives, Macadamia nuts, kale chips, dark chocolate, Greek yogurt, cheese in different forms, but also meat (as fresh as possible). You can also try naturally processed meat (without sulfites or sulfates) like deli, pepperoni, beef sticks and others.

Fasting for women

In general, when comparing men and women, women tend to burn more fat on a day-to-day basis and are more insulin sensitive than men. Women also have very different hormonal profiles. There are the obvious differences in sex hormones like testosterone and estrogen which affect not only our ability to burn fat and build muscle, but also influence where we store our body fat.

There are also large differences in some of the more important fat loss hormones. Men tend to have less circulating growth hormone than women, and women tend to have 2 to 3-times more leptin than men. A man's hormone levels also tend to be more stable than a woman's since many hormones tend to fluctuate within a women's menstrual cycle.

The fact that both leptin and growth hormone are higher in women may have to do with the higher estrogen levels found in women's bodies. It has been shown in healthy pre-menopausal and post-menopausal women that estrogen increases blood GH levels. In fact, the combination of high estrogen and high growth hormone is one of the hallmark hormonal markers of healthy young women. A healthy, young woman may secrete anywhere from 2 to 7-fold more GH than pre-pubertal girls, men, or post-menopausal women.

Because of these hormonal differences women will have higher amounts of free fatty acids in their blood compared to a man after longer periods of fasting (40 to 72-hours). These elevated levels of free fatty acids will cause a woman to remain in a heightened state of fat burning longer than a man for the period after the fast has been broken. This is evident by the increased fat oxidation even after a meal, slower glucose clearance, and the decreased ability for elevated insulin to push a woman out of fat burning during the hours following a fast.

So, it is true that women have a physiology that is uniquely their own, and many of these differences involve some of the most important fat-burning hormones. But how does this affect their ability to diet and lose unwanted body fat?

It is well known that prolonged food deprivation, large energy deficits created through vigorous exercise, and rapid weight loss all may result in various forms of menstrual dysfunction in some (but not all) women.

Or put differently, regardless of whether you are a man or a woman, young or old, bad things start to happen when your body fat levels become too low.

For men, the critical level of body fat seems to be closer to 4-6%,[259] but this also seems to vary slightly based on age and ethnicity. So, both men and women have healthy levels of body fat under which metabolic/ hormonal issues may arise, with the levels

For the vast majority of men and women, fasting once or twice a week for 24 hours combined with an exercise program and sensible eating is enough to cause significant weight loss, and maintenance of that weight loss. Adding in longer fasts, fasting more often, or excessively dieting on the days you are not fasting may not necessarily bring the results you think, or hope, it will.

Just like exercise or dieting, fasting can be overdone. For both men and women, the best advice I can give is to fit your fasting into your life, allow fat loss to happen at a natural pace (don't try to force it by combining fasting, dieting, and excessive exercise), and remember that the goal is NOT 0% body fat (neither for men nor for women).

Maintenance

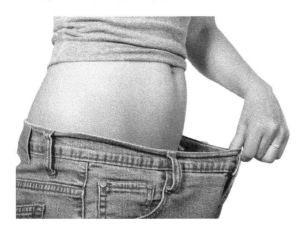

Maintaining Well-Balanced Meals

When following a fast, it's important that you're getting the right nutrition. If you don't want to follow a specific diet, then aim for healthy, wholesome foods. A good way of doing this is having a well-balanced meal.

Most of us have learned what a healthy meal constitutes in school. It was drilled into us during health class, possibly pointed to in biology class, and repeatedly mentioned by the school nurse. But most of us don't eat well-balanced meals. We instead eat what's convenient. With so many easy to find restaurants, food can be at our fingertips. Most of that food isn't healthy, and while it can be difficult for some Americans to find healthy foods, if you have them available to you, then choose wholesome foods, rather than fast foods.

If you have difficulty figuring out what makes a well-balanced meal, you can explore some of the resources provided by the U.S. Health Department. They even have a website dedicated to showing how to portion your meals and include all the food groups during your day. The website can offer you customizable meal plans that will give you nutritious meals and can provide other resources so that you can make the best meal decisions for your body type.

When you have a well-balanced meal, it means that you're eating a bit from at least three different food groups. The food groups are fruits, vegetables, grains, proteins, and dairy.

Fruit is...well...fruit. It's self-explanatory. While you want to eat some fruit each day, you're not going to eat as much as you do vegetables. Fruits can be high in sugar, so choose fruits that aren't as high and eat those more frequently. Try a variety of different kinds of fruit because they can each contain different vitamins and nutrients. So, pick and choose, and don't stick with the same fruit every day. Despite what they say, an apple a day doesn't keep the doctor away. Instead, mix up your fruit choices.

The vegetable family includes a lot of variety. Think pumpkins, corn, broccoli, onions, and beans. All of these are part of the vegetable group. They're also one of the largest families of food you should eat during your day. In general, at least one-third or half of your plate should be vegetables. Just like with fruit, you want to mix up your vegetables because they each provide a different type and number of vitamins. For example, yellow pumpkins can give you way more vitamin A than many other veggies. So, mix it up.

Grains are a large food group and the family consists of food produced by a grain plant. Some grain plants include wheat, bran, rye, rice, oats, and sometimes corn. All of this is then processed into other foods like bread, oatmeal, polenta, tortilla's, cereal, etc. All of these are a part of the grain food family. Grains should also be a large part of your meal. About one third of your plate will be grains. Whole grains are a better option than other types. Think whole-wheat bread vs. white bread. Choose brown rice over white rice. These types of grain contain more nutrients.

The protein family has a variety of different items in it. It can contain lean meats that are unprocessed, seafood, beans, nuts, and tofu. Some lean meats are lamb, beef, and pork. Sausages, hot dogs, and salami are considered processed and less healthy. You should eat these only in small quantities. But lean meat itself is quite healthy and you should eat about seven servings in a week. Seafood is another great choice and you should have at least two servings in your week. Seafood includes fish, shrimp, scallops, octopus, etc. Beans, nuts, and tofu are other kinds of protein. They are all plant based and are excellent alternatives to meat or seafood. You should try to have some meatless/plant-based foods during your week and beans can give you an alternative that will keep you full.

The dairy family is our last food group. It consists of animal products like milk, eggs, cheese, and yogurt. When you choose a dairy item, it should be a low-fat variety. Full fat yogurt can be very healthy and provide you with essential vitamins and probiotics. Dairy should only be a small percentage of your daily dietary consumption.

When choosing well-balanced meals, try to avoid heavily processed foods and fast foods. These can be full of sugar, carbs, and fats that aren't healthy for you. However, eating out every now and again is completely fine. Just don't make it a daily habit. Other foods like processed meats, alcohol, fatty foods, and 'junk' foods should be limited so that they do not take up a huge portion of your weekly eating.

While you fast, you want your food choices to give you the best balance of nutrients. So, following a well-balanced meal will help you maintain your weight, or even promote weight loss depending on what your diet was like before you started fasting. While you could eat all the right nutrients, you might still be sabotaging yourself with your portion sizes. So be aware of the portion size as well as the nutrients in each of your meals.

A lifestyle change

Obesity is not created by one specific macronutrient in our diet. In fact, it's not the diet at all. In my opinion, the number one cause of our obesity epidemic is abundance. There simply is too much food available for us to consume. Combine this with a highly effective and relentless food marketing industry and a misled and backwards health and nutrition industry and the problem becomes clear. Not only do most of us eat too much, but most of us have no idea why.

This is why Eat Stop Eat is not a diet; it is a lifestyle based on the nutritional custom of including the combination of short-term, flexible, and intermittent fasting along with resistance training into your life.

It's a way of life where you accept the idea of taking small 24-hour breaks from eating, and taking part in resistance exercises (working out with weights) at least two to three times a week. That's it. The Eat Stop Eat lifestyle is simply taking a 24-hour break from eating once or twice per week and a commitment to a workout routine.

All my research has led me to the conclusion that this is the single best and most uncomplicated way to lose weight, to maintain muscle, and to reap all the amazing health benefits associated with fasting. Keep in mind, brief breaks from eating are nothing new — almost all of us fast for 8 to 10 hours almost every night, so I'm simply asking you to expand this fast. It is also the easiest way to rid you of obsessive-compulsive eating and the need to constantly scour magazines and the internet for the latest and greatest diet strategy.

With Eat Stop Eat, you get rid of the compulsion and guilt that drives so many of today's eating habits, as we get rid of the idea that you need to be constantly eating, or that there is even one true "perfect" way to eat. The reason I don't consider this style of eating to be a diet is because unlike almost all popular diets, the Eat Stop Eat lifestyle is a sustainable addition to the way we eat for the rest of our lives.

Potential downsides

The risks you'll run into are bingeing, malnutrition, and difficulty with maintaining the fast. Suffice it to say, bingeing while you fast risks any of the benefits from fasting you might originally have. A bigger risk is malnutrition.

Malnutrition sounds alarming, but for the most part, you can prevent this by having well-balanced meals during your eating windows. The risk of malnutrition comes especially during the kinds of fast which include very low-calorie restriction on fasting days. If you're not eating the right nutrition throughout your week, the reduction in calories plus the poor nutrition can result in some of your dietary needs not being met. This could result in more weight loss, but also more muscle loss and other issues. To prevent this risk, you can ensure that your meals are nutritious and well-balanced. Have a variety of fruits and vegetables, try different meats and seafoods, and include grains unless you're following a specific diet like the keto diet.

Associated with malnutrition is dehydration. We get a lot of our daily water intake from the food we eat. But if you're eating a reduced amount of food during your day, or no food during your day, you're going to need to drink a lot more water than you normally do. If you're not keeping track of your hydration levels, it's possible for you to drink too little. To combat this risk, ensure that you're drinking enough by keeping a hydration journal. You could also track it in an app. Set up reminders to drink water and check your urine color. Light colored urine means good hydration, so check often despite how disgusting it might be to you.

Because fasting can be difficult to start, this can be one of the risks associated with it. You're going to feel hungry during the first couple weeks of following your fasting schedule. You may even feel uncomfortable, with mood swings, different bowel movements, and sleep disruptions. All of this can lead to you struggling with starting the fasts. They can also lead you to ignore greater warning signs that you shouldn't fast. These signs include changed heart rate, feelings of weakness, and extreme fatigue. These feelings shouldn't be ignored during the start. If you feel severely uncomfortable when you start your fast, you should stop and speak with your doctor.

The plan to getting started

When you have made the decision that this is something you want to try, you need to decide upon a starting date. You also need to make sure that all the temptations are removed from the fridge and that you don't have all the bad habit food left in the larder. It's a good idea to talk to people who are close to you so that they know you are embarking on this type of diet. That means that you will gain their support, and they will understand that between certain hours, you will not be permitted to eat. I find that people who do discuss the diet with family succeed because they gain more support. That helps them to keep to the times specified at the beginning of the fasting process.

The first night will be a little hard. People will offer you food after eight because they won't yet be accustomed to your dietary regime. If you find that you are distracted by people offering you food, use this time to introduce yourself to meditation or relaxation. This is excellent for you and will help you through difficult times. To relax, for example, lie down on the bed and close your eyes. Imagine each part of your body tensing up and then relaxing and you will find that time passes very quickly. Even if you decide to go to bed early with a book, you will get accustomed to this new lifestyle very soon.

Midday the first day

Just because midday has arrived, don't be tempted to eat more than you normally would. This is just the start of another cycle in your diet. It isn't an opportunity to eat loads of good things. If you have the energy, go for a walk before you eat because that will also help all of the calories that you eat to be used up. Then, when you eat, take the time to eat. As eating is important to you, chew your food correctly and try not to swallow your food too quickly. This also helps the digestive system to cope with this new onslaught of food.

Try to get out of the habit of drinking with your food. It's much better to take a drink after the meal. This helps digestion as well.

The afternoon

Try some healthy snacks during the afternoon. Instead of eating chocolate bars and drinking copious amounts of coffee, try to be inventive and find snacks that are healthy. There are loads of alternatives. You don't have to be on a strict diet, but if you want to see a difference soon, then being sensible about your foods will help this to happen.

The evening

Since you are usually going to give more time to your evening meal, and it's likely to be the biggest meal of the day, exercise before eating is a good way to ensure that the body is ready for the food being given to it. Then, when you sit down to eat your meal, enjoy every bit of it because that's the last food you will have for the next 24 hours. Enjoy the tastes and flavors and take your time eating your food, knowing that this helps the digestion.

Each night, after your meal, make sure that you keep a journal and in this journal put your progress. This can include your weight, your feelings, what new foods you have discovered or how you think you could improve your diet tomorrow. The journal is your reinforcement that the regime is working, and gradually you will begin to see a difference in your appearance that is pleasing. Your waistline, for example, may begin to slim down. You may find that you don't feel sluggish and that you have loads more energy. Write down all of the positive effects of your diet because this will help to spur you on when you have days with little enthusiasm.

You need to remind yourself of why you are doing this. You want to live longer, and you want the quality of your life to be better. That's enough incentive to stick to the new lifestyle, and you will soon be at a stage where you accept this as being your normal way of life. I would never go back to the way I was and feel healthier and fitter because of it.

Chapter 3: Benefits

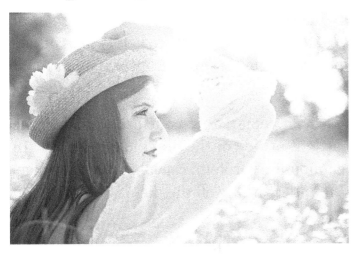

Benefits for weight loss

Obviously, the goal of any weight loss program should not be quick, short-lived weight loss. To truly reap the benefits of any weight loss program the results need to be long lasting. Let's face it, nobody wants to put the effort into losing weight just so they can gain it back. Typically, maximal weight loss occurs during the first 6 months of a diet, after which, weight regain slowly begins to set in. Luckily this could be one of the greatest strengths of Eat Stop Eat. Let me explain.

Most research looking at long-term weight loss follows a protocol like this: get a bunch of people and make them lose weight very quickly using a very-low-calorie diet with lots of clinical supervision, rules, support groups, follow up meetings, guidelines, and checklists.

Typically, once the subjects have lost roughly 10% to 15% of their original bodyweight they go on to the weight maintenance period of the study where researchers test different ways of eating to see if some are better than others at helping people maintain or even improve upon their weight loss.

The studies have been remarkably conclusive in that the specific macronutrient profile of the diet did not matter. In other words, the amount of protein, carbohydrates, and fats in the diet does not affect how well the diet is able help you keep the weight off.

In fact, research has found two things:

Your ability to keep the weight off is directly related to your ability to maintain a flexible amount of dietary restraint.

Your ability to keep the weight off is directly related to how well you maintained your lean body mass while you were losing weight.

Now, after reading point two you may immediately be thinking of some scientific explanation that includes the so-called "metabolism boosting" effect of lean mass. There is another just as plausible explanation to why preserving your lean body mass helps people lose weight. People will be rewarded psychologically and socially from the changes they've made in their body and be more willing to maintain dietary restraint in order keep this new body shape! In other words, having less fat and a defined lean body makes you look good, and it only takes a few compliments on your new lean toned body to keep you highly motivated to keep it up.

Regardless of why maintaining your lean body mass improves your ability to keep the weight off, the point remains: if you can follow a method of eating that allows you to eat less for long periods of time while still eating the foods you enjoy, and if you can preserve your lean body mass while you lose body fat, you greatly increase your chances of keeping the weight off!

This is the major benefit of Eat Stop Eat. You still eat the foods you like without restricting yourself to lists of good foods and avoiding everything on a list of bad foods. You still have to eat less, but you are in charge of the foods you choose to eat.

By being flexible and not restrictive, it allows you to enact a great deal of dietary restraint without feeling deprived or bored of your food choices. And a very large body of research suggests that this flexibility is a key to long-term weight loss success.

Other benefits

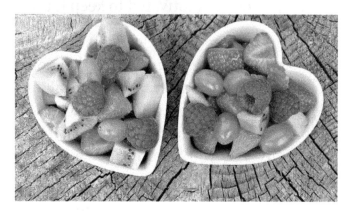

Benefits for hearth

At the time of this writing, heart problems are the number 1 cause of deaths worldwide. And when it comes to risks of heart problems, there are several health markers – a.k.a. Risk factors – that are linked to such risks. Intermittent fasting has been shown in several studies to improve several risk factors for heart problems like:

– Blood pressure;

– Blood sugar levels;

– Inflammation;

– Total and bad (LDL) cholesterol levels; and

– Triglycerides.

The only limitation to the studies that have noted these results is that most of them were conducted on animals. As such, more human studies must be conducted to reinforce these observed benefits of intermittent fasting.

Benefits for brain

Often times, things that benefit the body also benefit the brain. Another benefit associated with intermittent fasting is improvement of different metabolism-related things that may be considered crucial for brain health. These include lower blood sugar levels, lower insulin resistance, reduced inflammation, and less oxidative stress.

In several rat studies, intermittent fasting has been shown to help increase new nerve cell growth, which can be very beneficial for brain health and performance. I.F. was also shown to help raise BDNF, a.k.a. brain-derived neurotrophic factor, levels in the brain. When there's not enough BDNF, the risks of brain problems like depression are much higher. In other animal studies, intermittent fasting was also shown to be beneficial when it comes to protecting a person's brain from serious injuries due to strokes.

Chapter 4: The food on eat stop eat

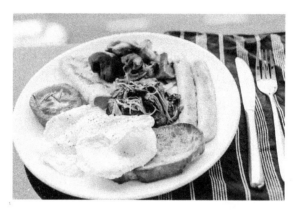

What should I eat?

I would stress the fact that on any diet, you need to avoid processed foods. You should aim for fresh produce, you are going to benefit more from fasting faster. Processed foods contain a multitude of ingredients that are not good for the body. Excess sodium, too much fat and certainly too much sugar are responsible for many serious ailments. They are also usually stripped of Fiber and contain little to no Micro-nutrients. You need to have a sensible approach to your diet so that when you do eat, you eat great food. That doesn't mean that everything has to be bland.

A combination of Beans and Rice or Mycoprotein are good for the body and provide you with your much-needed protein. If you aren't Vegan or Vegetarian and you do not want to choose a primarily Plant Based diet, you will have a few more obstacles but it isn't impossible for you to follow fasting. There are plenty of lean animal proteins on the market, choose whichever you prefer. For those who do not drink milk or who avoid dairy, whatever substitute you use must be natural, rather than heavily processed. I usually make my own Almond Milk and I buy Hemp Milk (it's the best). It's not going to be very good for you to replace natural foods with foods that are not natural, so be aware of the difference. Processed foods are your biggest enemy.

You can eat salads with dressings, and you can certainly eat sauces, but homemade sauces are always going to be preferable to those which are bought and which contain high quantities of sugar. When you go on an intermittent fasting regime, there are no real rules except for common sense. If you were to eat cakes and stodge all day, then it would certainly take more than 24 hours for your body to recover, so you need to be sensible in your approach. If you can avoid carbs which are considered as bad carbs, you will find that the results you want will happen quicker. Carbohydrates have quite a bad reputation, and this isn't always justified. However, if you use common sense, you will know that the carbs to avoid are those that are contained in cakes, biscuits, white bread etc. and that you need to replace bad carbs with good ones.

Thus, if you eat something along the lines lentils with a delicious salad, you are doing your body a favor as opposed to eating breaded fish and French fries. If you must eat French fries, at least use the oven baked fries that have hardly any fat content or invest in a fryer that prepares food with the minimum of fat. Fat is one of your worst enemies. You need to go over to using Olive Oil instead because this isn't a saturated fat. Or if you can afford it, I would suggest Safflower Oil, it can be a bit hard to find though. Similarly, instead of eating butter, why not switch to an Omega type spread? You will be cutting down on bad fats if you do and that helps your body to avoid the production of cholesterol. You need to look at the foods that you eat in a common sense manner. It isn't enough to simply starve yourself during the fast and then eat all of your favorite foods the moment you can. This has to be a life-changing event that helps you long term, rather than a short-term fad that merely helps you lose a few pounds. For the Omnivorous types, keep away from processed meats for the same reason as these contain too much bad fat. Snap away from that Slim Jim!

Fresh fruit is healthy, but be aware that an excess of fruit without Fiber will cause you to store the excess sugar as fat. Try to be reasonable in your consumption and avoid drinking juice since this is known to have a lot of sugar content with little fiber (unless you keep the pulp). If you do want to drink it, make sure that you have plenty of vegetables in the juice. Most vegetables contain significantly less sugar than their fruity counterparts and can still pack a tasty punch.

As long as you balance your diet and make sure that you eat regularly, you will lose weight, although the thing I found most beneficial was eating more often smaller portions instead of having a time of the day when I ate a hefty amount of food. My main meal was at seven in the evening – knowing that I would not be eating from 8 onward, but what I did to counter the effects of eating was exercise before the meal – so that my body was ready to digest the amount of food that made up my main meal.

If you love your coffee, then try to drink it without milk if you can get used to it. It certainly helps weight loss. If you must insist on using milk, try half fat or Almond milk because all of the fats that you feed your body have to be used up before weight loss occurs, and you may just be stopping yourself in your tracks if you overload on full cream milk, even if it is vegan. A sensible diet is required, but I also found that being adventurous gave me a lot more choices. I tried vegetables I had never eaten before and new fruits and found that foods such as asparagus became something that was incorporated more frequently, rather than turning to the comfort foods I had become accustomed to eating.

Cutting down on carbs

Sometimes, I wonder what is more dangerous to our bodies? Is it drugs, alcohol, tobacco? Well, I'm inclined to say that carbs are the most nocive to our bodies, especially that specific sub-group we also know as sugar. In some countries, there are extra fees for added sugar, so many drinks or products with excessive amounts of sugar cost more. By the way, have you looked recently at a bottle of Coca-Cola (or Pepsi), to see how much sugar it has? If not, then you might want to know that around 40% of the ingredients in those drinks is sugar.

This might make you think again about drinking (or giving to your children) any sodas, energy drinks, or normal natural juices (most of them have additional sugar, so it's not just fresh-squeezed juice). It's really hard to think that natural juice can only expire in a few months and no preservatives or special chemicals were added. Truth be told, every food or drink that is industrially processed can contain a high percentage of carbs. Even food that we consider normal can have a very high concentration of carbs. They can be found in bread, pastries, pasta, potatoes, rice, and many other products that are highly processed.

Pizzas or any other form of junk food have abundant carbs, so you might want to think again when eating all this food type. The problem with this food is that it has a very high-calorie level, but an extremely low nutrient value. Having just a burger with a soda next to eat is simply a caloric bomb, but guess what? You will feel hungry again in a short period; perhaps in less than 3 hours.

Sound familiar? Unfortunately, this type of food causes addiction, so as soon as you start feeling hungry again, your body will be craving for more carbs. Intermittent Fasting can help you control your calorie intake, but you need to make every calorie count, as you can't stuff your face with processed or junk food and expect to have results.

Therefore, you need to be very careful with your nutrition, and cutting down on carbs should be your starting point. You need to find out what food you need to avoid or to minimize the consumption of it. Therefore, this is what I'm suggesting: Try to eliminate the consumption of bread, pastry, and pasta (as much as possible)! Sorry, no sandwiches for you! Stay away from any fast-food place, and start eating more vegetables and fruits. You don't have to become vegan, but you need to carefully select the food you eat. Choose your own meal plan that best works for you!

If you don't have any idea about what you need to eat, try the Keto or the Mediterranean Diet! Since Intermittent Fasting is designed to make your body run on fats, basically making it the default "fuel," it's really important to keep eating fats. Now you are probably wondering: "But wait a minute! How can I eat fats and get slim?" Answering this question is really not complicated, as you stay away from glucose and carbs and keep fueling your body with fats to burn. Remember, Intermittent Fasting means also a lower calorie intake, so basically the fats you are eating should never have the chance to get stored in your fat tissue. Nutrition plays a very important role in the success of any IF program, so this one should make no exception. You can have a few normal days of eating, but try to make them matter and eat a lot healthier, and focus on having LCHF (Low Carbs High Fats) meal plans.

The importance of protein

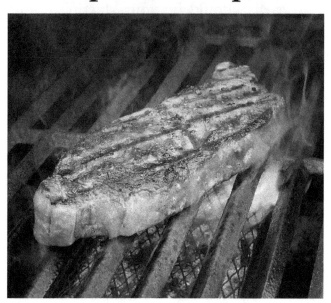

<u>Protein For Breakfast = Critical</u>

Although you're instructed to consume animal protein at "All Main Meals,' breakfast is by far the most important. Prioritizing animal protein at breakfast ensures a gradual and sustained increase in blood sugar, which means a consistent nutrient supply to the brain and the muscles. This not only keeps you satisfied longer, but it has a significant impact on the neurotransmitters that control hunger, brain function, metabolism, and overall energy levels. For instance, a study from the International Journal of Obesity in 2010 divided young students into 3 groups:

Skip Breakfast – 0g

Normal Protein – 18g

High Protein – 49g

It can be difficult to adjust to at first, but once you experience the increase in productivity and alertness they'll be no looking back. And experience with clients (from all walks of life) tells me that this one change can have the most profound effect on your results. The best strategy seems to be cooking extra dinner the night before and eating leftovers at breakfast; since most of us don't have time to put a steak on the BBQ at 6 in the morning.

Protein Improves Hormones

Animal Protein is the only food I classify as 'mandatory' because without it we may survive, but the long-term deterioration to our health, and increased risk of disease, make it impossible to thrive. As illustrated in **Eat Meat And Stop Jogging**, when we limit protein intake for the sake of calories our muscles suffer and so do our hormones. Ghrelin goes up and leptin goes down, which makes us consistently hungry and more likely to store what we consume as fat. And we experience significant muscle loss and a reduction in our metabolic rate, similar to what you'd expect with aging.

But that being said, filling up on animal protein is essential from a practical standpoint, because it's the best way to control hunger. Experience tells me that those who leave the house without eating breakfast, or don't have a plan for lunch or snacks throughout the day, set themselves up for failure.

No matter how disciplined you are, hunger finds a way to win in a head-to-head battle with the dessert bar in a coffee shop line.

Protein Promotes Fat Burning

Research has shown a direct correlation between the essential amino acids found in animal protein and one's ability to burn fat. A diet deficient in the amino acid Lysine has been tied to fat accumulation and fat in the liver, while a diet high in the amino acid Leucine associated with fat loss. Both amino acids must be present in order to experience these favorable results in body composition.

Whether or not it's the amino acids responsible for the fat loss, there's a considerable amount of scientific support suggesting that an increase in animal protein 'alone' promotes fat burning. For instance, a study from the journal of Nutrition and Metabolism gave one group of subjects 1.6g/kg bodyweight, and another 0.8g/kg, with an equal amount of daily calories. Although the weight loss was nearly equal, the high-protein group lost almost **entirely fat**.

When protein intake is adequate, fat loss is maximized without a reduction in muscle. In fact, when daily protein consumption is above average, there's the potential to gain muscle. This not only means a more attractive physique, but this translates to an increased metabolic rate, which means a higher daily burning rate.

By simply swapping a high-carb meal for a high-protein one, we experience a 100% greater increase in metabolism and this increase continues for 2.5hrs after eating!

When we consume animal protein regularly it has a profound effect on our body, as we burn **more** fat and build **more** muscle. And fortunately, your current body composition has no negative effect on whether or not your metabolic rate increases from a high protein meal. Meaning, there's still hope for individuals with a higher body fat to benefit just as much from the additional protein absorption and energy burning boost that comes with a high protein and low carbohydrate meal.

By making this minor adjustment a daily practice, we not only burn fat at a faster rate, but over-time we prevent the slow metabolic rate and muscle loss that's normally associated with aging.

Protein Supports Muscle

Research suggests that aging is associated with a reduction in muscle, which stems from a reduction in protein synthesis and absorption. As it turns out, the lowered protein absorption (or synthesis) seen in the elderly, is due to changes in the amount and activity of lean tissue. Meaning, the elderly have less muscle, and their bodies have a slower metabolic rate. Although many equate this physical outcome to 'aging,' research has proven that elderly with the same muscle as younger age groups absorb protein just as effectively. For instance, when you compare lean tissue pound-for-pound, as opposed to individuals with equal body weight, the absorption rates between the young and old are equivalent.

The lower protein absorption seen in the elderly has less to do with 'natural aging' and more to do with an inadequate intake of animal protein.

This was demonstrated nicely in a 2012 study in the European Journal of Applied Physiology where researchers originally found less muscle development from weight training in the elderly when compared to a younger age group over a 21-week training phase. What they later concluded, was that it wasn't because of greater synthesis or growth potential in the youth, but rather the old guys were barely consuming half the protein (0.8g/kg) of the young bucks (1.6g/kg).

Failure to facilitate muscle maintenance with nutritionally dense animal protein results in less muscle and a slower metabolism, especially as we age. Unfortunately, this is extremely common in the baby-boomer demographic, as this group has lived through the recommendations to eat low-fat, increase whole grains, do cardio, avoid saturated fat, restrict calories to lose, and limit meat to prevent cancer. Realistically:

Lower protein absorption is the result of less muscle and a slower metabolism; which is because of a restriction in animal protein, NOT because of age!

We must get essential amino acids from our diet, or we put our daily performance, body composition, and long-term health at risk. Largely because animal nutrition sources (meat, dairy, organ meats) are the only 'complete' proteins, which means they include all 9 essential amino acids. By consuming them on a daily basis, we not only give our body exactly what it needs, but we improve the bioavailability of these essential amino acids and facilitate muscle protein absorption. A biomarker that can drastically decline with age...if you let it!

Protein Supplies Essentials

Prioritizing protein is critical to supporting the needs of the musculoskeletal system. Failure to consume enough animal protein leads to muscle loss, which lowers your resting metabolic rate and weakens your structural frame. Calcium builds bone, but as we discussed in **Eat Meat And Stop Jogging**, the 'illusion of truth' is that additional dietary calcium means healthier bones. Unfortunately, extra dietary calcium does not add bone support if protein intake is too low. Furthermore, calcium absorption is largely dependent on Vitamin D, which is found primarily in animal protein. Older generations are not only at risk of falls and fractures due to an overall reduction in strength and muscle mass, but they generally fail to meet the animal protein requirement to maintain healthy bones.

Not Grains!

Similarly, as anthropologist, Mark Cohen discusses in his book 'Health and Rise of Civilization,' the strongest and healthiest lived in parts of Africa where there was the most 'Big Game.'

As in 'Big Large Animals to hunt.'

Although ketones are the driving fuel source in **Live It NOT Diet!**, protein and amino acids play a considerable role in determining our daily energy and wakefulness by activating key neurotransmitters in the brain. Not only stimulating them, but inhibiting any glucose that would otherwise block them.

Chapter 5: Exercise

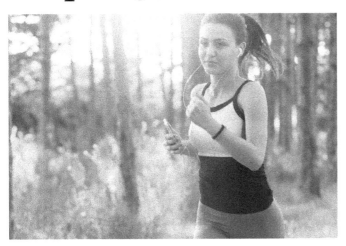

How exercise changes while fasting

The Eat-Stop-Eat can help you lose excess body fat and body weight. But as with any serious weight loss effort, combining a healthy and sensible fat-loss diet can help speed up the process. This is because it can help prevent or even speed up your metabolism and burn more body fat in the process. Resistance training exercises can help you preserve or even increase muscle mass, which is very important for a healthy metabolism.

Personally, I find that people who lose weight through a combination of diet and exercise tend to look better than people who lost weight through dieting alone. Those who include exercise in their weight loss strategy end up looking fitter and stronger compared to those that only diet. Hence, you should seriously consider incorporating regular exercise with the Eat-Stop-Eat protocol.

If you decide to incorporate regular exercise into your Eat-Stop-Eat, here are some practical tips for optimizing the benefits of regular exercise while fasting intermittently.

Optimal Timing

According to nutrition expert Christopher Shuff, you should ask yourself whether you should schedule your workouts before, within, or after your eating windows. To help you choose which time is the best time, you must think about what your goal is for exercising during your I.F.

If your primary goal is to burn as much body fat as possible, then try working out in a fasted state, i.e., 1 ½ hours before your eating window or at least 3 hours the window is optimal. Being in a fasted state will force your body to tap your glycogen and eventually, your body fat stores for energy during exercise. This optimizes fat-burning, but the trade-off is reduced physical performance, i.e., less weight lifted or lower exercise intensity.

But if your primary goal is optimal performance or strength and muscle building, you should schedule your workouts during your eating windows. Why? It's because you'll need all the easily accessible energy you can get to go all out on your workout sessions.

Another thing to consider is your own physical fitness level. If you're already used to performing physical exercises at a relatively high level even if you haven't eaten within 3 to 4 hours prior, i.e., a fasted state, then working out during your fasting days or before your eating window can be your best option for fat-burning. If you're not, then you'd be better off working out during your eating days.

Kinds of Workouts

Lynda Lippin, who's a certified personal trainer, says being cognizant of the calories or macronutrients you consumed the day prior to working out and those that you eat after. She says that if you want to do strength training exercises, you must make sure you get enough carbohydrates the day before and on the day of the workout itself. But if you plan to do cardio or high intensity interval workouts (HIIT), you can schedule it on days when you eat less carbohydrates.

Within the context of the Eat-Stop-Eat protocol and what Lippin said, you may be better off lifting weights during your eating days and doing steady state cardio or HIIT exercises during your fasting days for optimal fat-burning.

Post-Workout Nutrition

Scheduling your weight lifting or resistance training workouts during your regular eating days is optimal for fat-burning. This is because aside from having enough fuel to power your muscles for the heavy workload ahead, it also provides your muscles with much needed nutrients to avoid muscle catabolism. Remember, muscle catabolism can substantially slow down your metabolism. Hence, the need to avoid at all costs.

A good post-workout nutrition guide is to consume a good amount of carbohydrates, particularly starchy carbohydrates with around 20 grams of good quality protein after at least 1 hour. Why that long? According to top fitness and nutrition expert Shaun Hadsall of the Over 40 Ab Solution program, waiting for at least an hour after you end your exercise allows you to "ride" your body's fat-burning wave and burn more fat before you nourish your muscles with much-needed protein and glycogen.

Pre-Workout Nutrition

For optimal physical performance during your weight-lifting sessions, you'll need to ensure your body's glycogen stores are filled up. Doing so will ensure you have enough fuel to power through a very grueling weight-lifting session.

Hydration and Electrolyte Levels

When exercising, always keep a bottle of water close by so you can continually stay hydrated regardless if lifting weights at the gym on your eating days or doing steady state cardio on your fasting days. Ideally, drink between 17 to 20 ounces of water 2 to 3 hours prior to working out or doing steady state cardio and another 8 ounces 30 minutes prior. During exercise, drink between 7 and 10 ounces every 10 to 20 minutes. Post exercise drink another 8 ounces within 30 minutes.

If you're particular about maintaining good electrolyte levels, consider drinking fresh, plain coconut water. It's high in electrolytes but, unlike sports drinks like Gatorade, it is low in sugar and total calories, which makes it perfect for your fat-burning goals.

Intensity and Duration

When exercising during your fasting days, it's best to keep exercise duration and intensity between low to medium only. This is because you aren't getting any calories that day, which will make you significantly less strong with shorter stamina. If you push it to the hilt, you may feel dizzy or worse, faint from sheer exhaustion. That's why the best workout for your fasting days – should you decide to exercise – is low to medium intensity steady state cardio for up to 30 minutes maximum. Examples of low to moderate steady state cardio include brisk walking on the road or on a treadmill, leisurely biking around the neighborhood on relatively level ground, and stationary biking.

Pay Attention to Your Body

Your fasting day isn't the time to go all gung-ho by dismissing what your body's telling you, especially if it's telling you how bad it already feels. If you feel dizzy or weak, stop exercising. Chances are high that you're either dehydrated, low in blood sugar, or both. Drink lots of water and rest. If you still feel dizzy from hunger, don't be a martyr and insist on continuing your fast for that day. Ditch that day's fast, drink an electrolyte-rich drink and eat a healthy meal to normalize your blood sugar levels too. Sports drinks are okay in this situation, given your low electrolyte and blood sugar levels. Just learn your lesson and keep your cardio session levels to moderate at most and for 30 minutes maximum only on your succeeding fasting days.

Design your workout plan

In most research trials where people on a low-calorie diet preserved lean mass by using resistance training, their workouts fit into the following parameters: they typically worked out 3 to 4 times per week with each workout session lasting about 45 minutes. On average, 2 to 3 muscle groups would be exercised per workout session. Each workout consisted of between 6 to 10 exercises with each exercise being completed for 2 to 4 sets of 8 to 12 reps. Rest periods would consist of up to 2 minutes rest between each set of an exercise.

As an example, it takes a high amount of weight, volume, and stress for a 250-pound bodybuilder to maintain a high level of muscle mass. If a 250-pound bodybuilder were to follow Eat Stop Eat, the amount and type of exercise that he would need to do to maintain his muscle mass would be much greater than what a 145-pound woman who hasn't previously exercised would need to do. Further, a 145-pound woman who hasn't previously exercised in this manner would see very little benefit from immediately following the bodybuilder's workout routine.

Selecting the appropriate exercise program depends on the following factors:

Your current training status (how much you currently work out)

Your goals (maintain or gain muscle)

The amount of muscle mass you are currently carrying

An easy rule of thumb would be to look at the amount of exercise you were doing before you started following Eat Stop Eat, and make sure to slowly progress from there. Just like your nutrition program, your workout routine should revolve around the simplest and easiest methods that get you the results you want.

The Importance of Sticking with It

If you are fairly inactive, then starting a workout program may actually be very difficult. Research has suggested that as many as 50% of people who start a new exercise program will drop out within six months. Most of the time people say the reason that they stop exercising is that they are tired or because of lack of time. It is very important that you stick with your program, short of becoming obsessive about exercise.

Not only will sticking to your workout program help you preserve muscle mass while you are losing body fat, but it will also keep your mood elevated. In some very interesting research published in 2008, it was found that when a group of women who exercised regularly were forced to stop exercising for 72 hours, there was a noticeable decrease in their body satisfaction and mood.

The results of this study also showed that after 72 hours of non-exercise, feelings of tension, anxiety, and sluggishness were increased. Of course, this is ironic considering that these are the exact reasons why most people stop working out in the first place.

This leads to the idea of a downward spiral when you quit an exercise routine. You quit because you are tired or stressed, only to become even more tired and even more stressed, and then the spiral picks up momentum, and you end up glued to your couch unable to even think about the stress of restarting another exercise program.

When it comes to exercise, balance seems to be the key. Too much exercise and you increase the risk of overuse injuries and you could become obsessive, defining yourself as a person by your exercise program. Too little exercise and you lose the muscle maintaining and myriad of health benefits. Not only this, but you also run the risk of becoming dissatisfied with your body, as well as experience a decreased mood.

For Eat Stop Eat the goal is to use exercise as a tool. Doing the amount needed to preserve or build some muscle, but not becoming obsessive to the point where exercise interferes with your life. You should look forward to your next workout session, not dread it. And never let it define who you are as a person.

For this reason, I recommend keeping your exercise plans as uncomplicated as possible. Stimulate your muscle following the suggestion in the above paragraphs, allow them to recover, then repeat when you are ready.

Health benefits of exercise

Enhanced insulin sensitivity (which will help make fasting easier overall)

Build muscle quicker and more efficiently

Improve recovery time (with BCAA supplementation)

Better lifting via muscle glycogen retention and repletion

Improved adaption to exercise

No matter what your end goal is, exercise more. If you can, do it on an empty stomach. Period. Just be sure to drink plenty of water!

Chapter 6: Breakfast Recipes

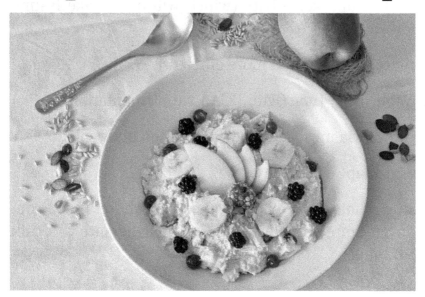

Crunchy Banana Yoghurt

Serves: 1

Ingredients:

• 6 ounces fat-free natural Greek yogurt

Toppings: Use any one or more

• 1 teaspoon pumpkin seeds

• 1 teaspoon sesame seeds

• 1 teaspoon sunflower seeds

• Toasted, slivered almonds

- 1 small banana sliced

Directions:

Add yogurt into a bowl. Place banana slices on top. Sprinkle the suggested toppings and serve.

Cinnamon Porridge with Grated Pear

Serves: 4

Ingredients:

- 4.5 ounces jumbo porridge oats

- 20 ounces semi-skimmed milk

- Juice of a lemon

- ½ teaspoon ground cinnamon + extra to garnish

- 2 ripe medium pears, peeled, cored, grated

Directions:

Add oats, milk and cinnamon into a non-stick saucepan. Place the saucepan over medium heat

Stir constantly until thick.

Divide into 4 bowls.

Top with grated pears. Drizzle lemon juice on top and serve.

Acai Smoothie Bowl

Serves: 2

Ingredients:

- 1 large bananas, sliced, frozen

- ¼ cup soy milk

- 7 ounces unsweetened acai berry pulp, frozen

For topping:

- 4 tablespoons granola

- 1 large banana, sliced

Directions:

Add banana, acai berry pulp and soy sauce into a blender and blend until thick and smooth.

Divide into 2 bowls. Top with banana slices and granola and serve.

Oatmeal Smoothie

Serves: 2

Ingredients:

- ½ cup old fashioned oats or quick oats

- 1 cup unsweetened almond milk

- 1 tablespoon pure maple syrup + extra to garnish

- 1 teaspoon ground cinnamon

- Ice cubes, as required, crushed (optional)

- 2 bananas, sliced, frozen

- 2 tablespoons creamy peanut butter

- 1 teaspoon pure vanilla extract

- ¼ teaspoon kosher salt

Directions:

Gather all the ingredients for smoothie. Set aside the ice and add the rest of the ingredients into a blender.

Blend for 30-40 seconds or until smooth. Add ice and pulse for a few seconds.

Pour into tall glasses and serve.

Peach, Raspberry and Nuts Smoothie

Serves: 1

Ingredients:

For smoothie:

- ½ cup fresh raspberries
- 1 peach, pitted, sliced
- 1mmedium banana, sliced
- ½ cup low fat yogurt
- 25-30 almonds, soaked in water for a few hours

For topping:

- 2-3 raspberries
- 2 soaked almonds, slivered
- 2-3 peach slices

Directions:

Gather all the ingredients for a smoothie and add into a blender.

Blend for 30-40 seconds or until smooth.

Pour into a tall glass. Add crushed ice if desired. Top with raspberries, almonds and peaches and serve.

Chapter 7: Lunch Recipes

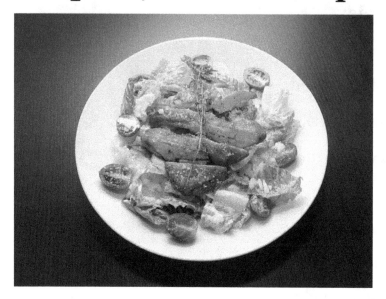

Easy Chicken Salad

Serves: 6

Ingredients:

Chicken Breast (1.5 pound)

Celery (3 stalks, sliced)

Mayo (0.5 cup)

Brown Mustard (2 teaspoons)

Salt (0.5 teaspoon)

Dill (2 tablespoons, fresh & chopped)

Pecans (0.25 cup, chopped)

Directions

Heat the oven to 425 degrees and line a baking sheet with parchment paper, aluminum foil, or baking spray.

Add chicken breast and cook until done throughout. This will take about 15 minutes.

Cool the breast completely. This can take anywhere from 10-30 minutes. Once cooled, cut into bite-size pieces.

Take a large-sized bowl and stir everything except the dill and pecans together.

Cover and chill about 1 hour before adding in dill and pecans. Serve cold.

Sautéed Mushrooms & Bacon with Greens

Serves: 2

Ingredients:

Bacon (4 slices, cut into half-inch pieces)

Mushrooms (2 cups, halved; your choice)

Salt (0.5 teaspoon)

Thyme (2 sprigs fresh herb, destemmed)

Garlic (3 cloves, minced)

Greens (2 cups; your choice)

Salad Dressing (0.25 cup; your choice)

Directions

Assemble the side-salad quickly by taking your choice of greens and sprinkling on a bit of dressing. Set aside or place in the refrigerator for just a few moments.

Take a large-sized skillet and bring to medium heat. Add bacon and cook until desired crispiness is reached. Stir in mushrooms and bring to browned color.

Stir in salt, thyme leaves, and garlic. Cook 5 minutes then serve hot alongside your salad.

Curry Chicken Half-Wraps

Serves: 2

Ingredients:

Chicken Thighs (1 pound, boneless & skinless)

Onion (0.25 cup, minced)

Garlic (2 cloves, minced)

Curry Powder (2 teaspoons)

Salt (1.5 teaspoons)

Butter (3 tablespoons)

Cauliflower Rice (1 cup)

Low-Carb Wraps (cut into halves)

Or lettuce leaves

Yogurt or Sour Cream (0.25 cup, for garnish)

Directions

Start by preparing your chicken thighs; cut them into one-inch pieces.

Take a large-sized skillet and heat 2 of the 3 tablespoons of butter on the skillet at medium heat. Add onion and cook till soft and browned.

Stir in chicken pieces, garlic, and salt. Cook for about 10 minutes.

Stir in the last tablespoon of butter, curry powder, and cauliflower rice. Cook about 5 minutes longer.

Serve in lettuce leaves or half-wraps, and top with a scoop of cream! Enjoy.

Pulled Pork Sliders

Serves: 4

Ingredients:

Pork Roast (3 pounds, boneless, cut into inch pieces)

Butter (1 tablespoon)

Salt (2 teaspoons)

Garlic Powder (2 teaspoons)

Onion Powder (1 teaspoon)

Black Pepper (1 teaspoon)

Smoked Paprika (1 tablespoon)

Tomato Paste (2 tablespoons)

Apple Cider Vinegar (0.5 cup)

Coconut Aminos (2 tablespoons)

Bone Broth (0.5 cup)

Butter (0.25 cup, melted)

Directions

Trim any fat from your pork roast and then cut it into appropriate chunks.

In a small-sized bowl, combine salt, paprika, pepper, onion and garlic powders and then rub the mixture onto the pork.

Grab a large-sized skillet and melt the tablespoon of butter before adding your chunks of pork to the skillet as well.

In a separate, medium-sized bowl, combine all other ingredients and pour over the pork in the skillet.

Boil the mixture to start then simmer for 30 minutes until meat is tender and is easy to pull apart in the sauce.

Serve on low-carb bread alternative or eat in portions alone.

Chapter 8: Dinner Recipes

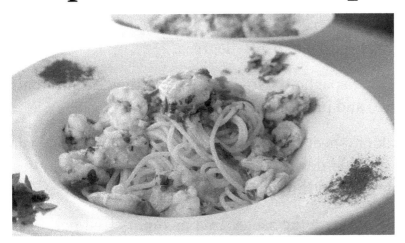

Unforgettable Spaghetti Squash

Serves: 4

Ingredients:

Spaghetti Squash (1 medium-sized OR equivalent of 3 pounds)

Garlic (3 cloves, minced)

Olive Oil (1 teaspoon)

Spinach (half-pound, chopped)

Heavy Cream (0.5 cup)

Parmesan Cheese (0.5 cup)

Salt & Pepper (to taste)

Mozzarella (grated for topping)

Directions

First, preheat the oven to 400 degrees.

Prepare the spaghetti squash by cutting it in half (lengthwise) and pulling out any seeds.

Line a baking sheet or grease it and lay spaghetti squash with the cut side down on the sheet. Roast 30-40 minutes until easily stabbed through with a fork.

Meanwhile, prepare the sauce. In a medium-sized pot, heat olive oil and garlic for no more than 5 minutes. Stir in spinach, cream, and parmesan in turn.

Season with salt and pepper and set aside.

When squash has finished roasting, pull it out from oven and begin to pull apart the strands of the squash itself (its name should make sense to you now if it didn't already!).

With the squash threads freed, pour the cheese mixture onto the squash and into the inner "boat" part. Top with extra parmesan and mozzarella, as desired, then bake at 350 degrees for 20 additional minutes.

At the last second, switch oven to broil and bring cheese to a beautiful browned color. Enjoy hot!

Parmesan Bacon-Asparagus Roll-Ups

Serves: 2

Ingredients:

Maple-Flavored Syrup (0.5 cup)

Butter (0.5 cup)

Salt (0.5 teaspoon)

Black Pepper (0.25 teaspoon)

Asparagus (2 pounds, washed & ends removed)

Bacon (8 slices, thick bacon)

Parmesan (2 tablespoons + 2 teaspoons, grated)

Directions

Start by preheating oven to 425 degrees.

Then, grab a small-sized pot and bring it to medium-low heat on the stove top. Add syrup, butter, salt, and pepper. Whisk together until smooth and heated through. Set aside for later.

Divide your 2 pounds of asparagus into 8 equal-sized groups. Wrap each group with a strip of bacon and secure the ends with toothpicks, as needed.

Line greased baking sheet with asparagus/bacon bundles then pour over with syrup mixture and half the parmesan.

Bake in the oven for 30 minutes. Then, switch to broil and bring the rack to the top shelf of the oven.

Broil 2 minutes until crispy and partially-charred.

Serve with toothpicks removed and enjoy!

Salmon Seared with Light Cream Sauce

Serves: 6

Ingredients:

Olive Oil (2 tablespoons)

Salmon Fillets (3, 6-ounce fillets)

Garlic (2 cloves, minced)

Light Cream (1 cup)

Cream Cheese (1 ounce)

Capers (2 tablespoons)

Lemon Juice (1 tablespoon)

Dill (2 teaspoons, fresh OR 1 tablespoon, dried)

Parmesan Cheese (2 tablespoons, grated)

Directions

Grab a medium-sized skillet and heat the oil to start. Add the salmon fillets once heated through and cook 5 minutes on each side.

Set fish aside to get the sauce together.

In that same pan, add garlic and cook on medium heat for 2 minutes. Add cream, cream cheese, lemon juice, and capers. Simmer for 5 minutes or until thickened.

Once thickening begins, return salmon to pan and spoon the sauce over each of the fillets.

On low heat now, bring the salmon to the appropriate temperature. Garnish with dill and parmesan and serve!

Single-Pan Fajita Steak

Serves: 5

Ingredients:

Garlic (2 cloves, minced)

Onion (1 medium-sized, sliced thinly)

Chili Powder (1 teaspoon)

Cumin (1 tablespoon)

Salt & Pepper (to taste)

Coconut Oil (0.25 cup)

Lime (1, juiced & zested)

Lemon (1, juiced & zested)

Steak (1 pound, sliced into strips)

Red Pepper (1 large-sized, sliced into strips)

Yellow Pepper (1 large-sized, sliced into strips)

Directions

Prepare the meat and vegetables and then stir all ingredients together on a lined or greased baking sheet.

Preheat oven to 350 degrees then bake for 15 minutes. Half-way through the process, stir the mixture well.

Serve with an extra sprinkle of lime juice.

Chapter 9: Dessert Recipes

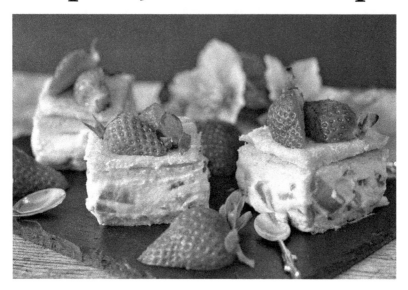

Chilled Cream

Serves: 8

Ingredients:

2-cans (15-oz.) coconut milk, refrigerated for at least 3 hours

2-cups heavy cream

1-tsp pure vanilla extract

¼-cup sweetener

A pinch of kosher salt

Directions:

1. Spoon the refrigerated coconut milk into a large bowl. Leave the liquid in the can. By using a hand mixer, beat the milk until turning creamy. Set aside.

2. Beat the heavy cream in a separate large bowl until it forms soft peaks. Add the vanilla and sweetener. Beat again until fully combined.

3. Fold in the whipped milk into the whipped cream. Mix well and transfer the mixture in a loaf pan.

4. Place the pan in the freezer for 5 hours until the mixture becomes solid.

Carrot Compact Cake

Serves: 2

Ingredients:

1-block (8-oz.) cream cheese, softened

¾-cup coconut flour

1-tsp sweetener

½-tsp pure vanilla extract

1-tsp cinnamon

¼-tsp ground nutmeg

½-cup pecans, chopped

1-cup carrots, grated

1-cup unsweetened coconut, shredded

Directions:

1. Combine the first six ingredients in a large mixing bowl. Mix well by using a hand mixer until fully combined. Fold in the pecans and carrots.

2. Form 16 balls from the mixture, and roll each ball in shredded coconut.

Choco Coco Cookies

Serves: 3

Ingredients:

¼-cup coconut oil

4-tbsp butter, softened

2-tbsp sweetener

4-pcs egg yolks

1-cup dark unsweetened chocolate chips

1-cup coconut flakes

¾-cup roughly chopped walnuts

Directions:

1. Preheat your oven to 350°F. Line a baking tray with parchment paper.

2. Combine all the ingredients in a large mixing bowl stir togetheregg yolks, sweetener, butter, and coconut oil. Mix in chocolate chips, coconut, and walnuts. Mix well until fully combined.

3. Form cookies out of the mixture, and place them in the baking tray. Bake for 15 minutes until golden.

Butter Ball Bombs

Serves: 3

Ingredients:

½-tsp. pure vanilla extract

½-tsp. kosher salt

8-tbsp (1 stick) butter

⅓-cup sweetener

2-cups almond flour

⅔-cup unsweetened dark chocolate chips, dairy-free

Directions:

1. By using your hand mixer, beat the butter in a large bowl until light and fluffy. Add the sweetener, vanilla extract, and salt. Beat again until fully combined.

2. Add gradually the almond flour, beating continuously until no dry portions remain. Fold in the chocolate chips. Cover the bowl with a plastic wrap and refrigerate for 20 minutes to firm slightly.

3. By using a small spoon, scoop the dough to form into small balls.

Choco 'Cado Twin Truffles

Serves: 3

Ingredients:

1-cup melted dark chocolate chips, dairy-free

1-pc small avocado, mashed

1-tsp vanilla extract

¼-tsp kosher salt

¼-cup cocoa powder

Directions:

1. Combine the melted chocolate with avocado, vanilla, and salt in a bowl. Mix well until fully combined. Refrigerate for 20 minutes to firm up slightly.

2. By using a small spoon, scoop about a tablespoon of the chocolate mixture and roll it in the palm of your hand to form a ball. Repeat the process to consume the mixture.

3. Roll each ball in cocoa powder.

Chapter 10: Snack Recipes

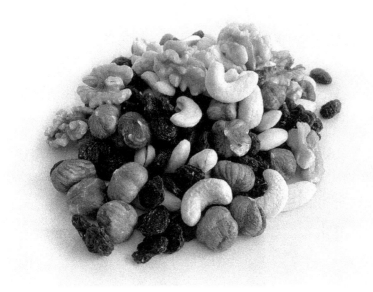

Kale Chips

Serves: 2

Ingredients:

Salt (1 tsp.)

Lime juice (2 Tbsp.)

Zest of a lime (1 pc.)

Sriracha (1 tsp.)

Olive oil (0.25 c.)

Cooking spray

Torn kale (1 bag)

Pepper (0.5 tsp.)

Directions

Preheat the oven to 400 degrees. Take out two baking pans and coat them with some cooking spray.

In a large bowl, whisk together the black pepper, salt, lime zest and juice, sriracha, and olive oil.

Take out the torn kale, add it to the bowl, and then toss until the leaves are coated with the dressing.

Spread the kale onto single, even layers on the baking sheet.

Bake in the oven for about 10 minutes, or until the kale is crisp. You can take the chips out of the oven and allow them to cool off.

Cinnamon Cocoa Popcorn

Serves: 4

Ingredients:

Cinnamon (1 tsp.)

Cocoa powder (1 Tbsp.)

Cooking spray

Popcorn kernels (0.5 c.)

Coconut oil (3 Tbsp.)

Salt (1 tsp.)

Sugar (1 Tbsp.)

Directions

Take out a one-gallon pot and heat up three tablespoons of coconut oil on medium-high. Add popcorn kernels one by one, and then when one of the kernels start to pop, you know that it is hot enough. Add in the rest of the kernels.

Cover the pot with the lid and shake the pot vigorously and frequently to make sure that there isn't any burning. When the popcorn is popped, you can move the popcorn to a mixing bowl.

First, make sure your hands are clean, then spray your popcorn with some cooking spray. Using your hands, toss the popcorn to mix well.

Sprinkle with the salt, sugar, cinnamon, and cocoa powder. Make sure that the popcorn is coated properly before serving.

Trail Mix

Serves: 2

Ingredients:

Sunflower seeds (2 Tbsp.)

Dark chocolate chips (3 Tbsp.)

Dried tart cherries (3 Tbsp.)

Dried apricots (10 pcs.)

Raw almonds (0.5 c.)

Directions

To get make your trail mix, add the almonds, sunflower seeds, chocolate chips, cherries, and apricots to a bowl.

Toss all these together and then add it to a resealable container. You can store this mix for up to 1 month.

Orange and Apricot Bites

Serves: 3

Ingredients:

Coconut (0.66 c.)

Almond butter (0.5 c)

Dried apricots (0.5 c.)

Pitted dates (1.5 c.)

Rolled oats (1 c.)

Vanilla (1 tsp.)

Orange juice (3 Tbsp.)

Zest of an orange (1 Tbsp.)

Directions

Preheat the oven to 350 degrees and line some parchment paper on a baking sheet. Place the oats on the baking sheet and toast them for a few minutes until they are slightly toasted.

While your oats are in the oven, take out the food processor and add in the dates. Pulse until smooth.

Add the vanilla, orange juice and zest, coconut, almond butter, apricots, and toasted oats to the food processor.

Pulse so that the mixture becomes a smooth consistency. Move contents into a bowl.

Use your hands to make little balls out of the batter and place them into a resealable container. Allow these to set for at least 15 minutes and then serve.

Peanut Butter Energy Cookies

Serves: 3

Ingredients:

Peanut butter, creamy (0.5 c.)

Salt (0.25 tsp.)

Baking soda (1 tsp.)

Cocoa powder (0.25 c.)

Flour (1 c.)

Chopped peanuts (0.5 c.)

Rolled oats (2 c.)

Vanilla (1 tsp.)

Beaten eggs (2 pcs.)

Brown sugar (0.5 c.)

Milk (0.5 c.)

Greek yogurt (0.25 c.)

Mashed banana (1 c.)

Directions

Using a bowl, sift together the salt, baking soda, cocoa powder, and flour.

In another bowl, mix together the milk, Greek yogurt, banana, and peanut butter. Add the brown sugar and then stir to combine. Finally, add the vanilla and the eggs and combine.

Next, add the flour to the peanut butter mixture along with the oats and peanuts. Stir well until a uniform moist consistency is reached. Cover the bowl and place in the fridge for 30 minutes.

Preheat the oven to 350 degrees, take out two baking sheets, and coat them with cooking spray.

Place a spoonful of the batter onto the baking sheet for each cookie, making sure to leave plenty of space between each. You should be able to fit around twelve cookies per sheet. Use a fork to press them down a little bit, giving the cookies the usual crisscross pattern. Place in the oven to bake.

After about 15 minutes, you can take the cookies out of the oven and allow them to cool down before serving.

CONCLUSION

The health problems caused by today's nutrition are profound. Things have changed dramatically over the last decades, and more and more people are now suffering from diabetes (or other diseases related to high blood sugar and pressure), and the number of deaths caused by them has multiplied significantly. Clearly, something has to change in order to put an end to this madness, and the info and tips provided by this book can help you improve your health, physical fitness and wellbeing. Intermittent Fasting can be the solution you need, and if you want to try the Eat Stop Program, I would encourage you to read Brad Pilon's book "Eat Stop Eat," in addition to the tips in this book. If you had an "epiphany" and want to change your life by following the guidelines mentioned in this book, let me congratulate you and thank you for reading this book. You have chosen one of the most sustainable and revolutionary way to lose weight and improve your health.

CPSIA information can be obtained
at www.ICGtesting.com
Printed in the USA
LVHW040352091020
668360LV00001B/64